Leaner, Stronger, Smarter for life

Gain Muscle, Lose Fat, Keep It Off

by

Mikael Andersson

Dear reader,

Welcome to "Leaner, Stronger, Smarter for life Gain Muscle, Lose Fat, Keep It Off" With over 30 years of experience as a sports nutritionist and personal trainer, I've witnessed firsthand the transformative power of a well-structured nutrition and training plan. This book is your guide to understanding and implementing the principles that will help you achieve and maintain your health and fitness goals for life.

Contrary to common misconceptions, lifting weights isn't just for those looking to "bulk up." It's a fundamental component of a balanced fitness regimen, essential for maintaining muscle mass and keeping fat at bay, especially after a diet. However, dieting alone falls short without incorporating strength training to support your body's composition and overall health.

This book is designed not only for those aiming to lose weight or gain muscle but for anyone serious about improving their health and fitness. Through the pages of this guide, you'll discover practical advice, backed by scientific research and decades of experience, to help you build a lifestyle that supports your fitness journey every step of the way.

Whether you're just starting out or looking to refine your approach to nutrition and training, this book offers insights into creating a balanced, sustainable plan that works for you. Let's embark on this journey together, towards a healthier, stronger life.

Mikael Andersson is a seasoned sports nutritionist and personal trainer with over 30 years of experience in the field. With a lifelong passion for health and fitness, Mikael has dedicated his career to helping individuals achieve their optimal physical condition through personalized nutrition and training programs. His holistic approach to fitness has transformed the lives of thousands, guiding them towards a healthier, more fulfilling lifestyle.

Table of Contents

Introduction

Are you one of those people who are striving to achieve a healthier, fitter, and stronger body, but feeling overwhelmed by the conflicting information and the complexities of human physiology? The path to fitness may seem daunting, but the principles governing muscle gain and fat loss are based on science, and when understood, they can help you transform your body.

This book is not just another superficial guide that promises quick fixes and fad diets. It demands a foundational change in lifestyle, a deep understanding of the science behind body transformation, and the mental fortitude to overcome challenges. By combining instructtional guidance, scientific insights, and motivational strategies, this book aim to equip you with the tools to initiate and sustain this transformative journey.

The objective is not just to help you lose weight but to guide you in reshaping your physique through muscle gain and fat loss, achieving a healthier and more vibrant version of yourself. The basic principles of body composition, including the roles that muscle mass and fat play in metabolism, are crucial to understanding the science behind body recomposition. This book highlights these concepts while debunking common misconceptions that could derail your progress.

With scientific evidence at its backbone, the content spans from the macro to micro aspects of body recomposition, covering everything from the overarching concepts of energy balance to the specifics of nutrition, strength training, cardiovascular exercise, and recovery practices. But, it don't just stop there. This book take you beyond the basics and delve into how you can tailor nutrition and training routines to your unique physiological makeup, lifestyle, and goals. This individualized approach ensures that the strategies you adopt are sustainable in the long run, paving the way for not just temporary changes, but a lifetime of wellness and strength.

In summary, this book is a comprehensive guide for anyone looking to embark on a transformative fitness journey. Whether your goal is to shed a significant amount of body fat, gain muscle mass, or both, the evidence-based strategies and motivational insights within these pages will serve you on your journey. So, are you ready to transform your body, grounded in the science of body recomposition, fueled by a steadfast commitment, and inspired by the limitless potential of the human body? Let's begin this journey together!

Chapter 1:
Understanding Body Composition

Starting this journey towards better health and fitness begins with a foundational understanding of your body's composition. It's an enlightening first step that paves the way for effective fat loss and muscle gain, guiding you to results that are not only desirable but sustainable. Body composition, reflecting the proportion of fat and muscle in your body, serves as a more comprehensive indicator of health than weight alone. Delving into the science of body composition, it becomes clear that the interplay between muscle mass and body fat is intricate, with each component playing an important role in metabolism.

Muscle mass plays a vital role in our body's strength and stamina, and not just in burning calories. On the other hand, body fat is essential for hormone regulation and energy storage, so it's important to aim for a healthy balance rather than just focusing on weight loss. There are many misconceptions about body composition, from the idea that muscle can turn into fat to the belief that fat loss can be targeted. However, understanding and embracing the complexities of your body composition can lead to a significant and long-lasting transformation, resulting in improved health and fitness for life.

It's important to remember that achieving a healthy body is not just about the numbers on a scale. It's about understanding what those numbers represent and how they can affect your overall health. By balancing muscle and fat, you can greatly improve your metabolic health, physical appearance, and overall wellbeing. As you move forward towards your goals, keep in mind that reshaping your body composition is a powerful way to unlock your full potential. This means not only achieving a leaner physique, but also experiencing a more energetic and vibrant life.

The Basics of Body Fat, Muscle Mass, and Their Roles in Metabolism

Understanding body fat and muscle mass, as well as their roles in metabolism, is fundamental to getting a grasp on overall health, fitness, and the body's energy systems.

Body Fat: Body fat, or adipose tissue, plays several crucial roles in the body:

Energy Storage: Fat is a dense source of energy, providing about 9 calories per gram. It serves as a vital energy reserve for the body during times of need. **Protection and Insulation:** Fat cushions and protects vital organs and helps maintain body temperature by providing insulation. **Hormone Regulation:** Adipose tissue secretes hormones and other substances that influence metabolism, appetite, and the function of other organs. Body fat percentage is a common way to assess an individual's fitness level and health risks, with recommended ranges varying by age, sex, and fitness level.

Muscle Mass Muscle mass refers to the weight of muscle in your body. Muscles are made up primarily of protein and water and serve several key functions:

Movement and Strength: Muscles generate force and movement, enabling physical activity and bodily functions. **Metabolism:** Muscle tissue is metabolically active, meaning it burns calories even at rest. More muscle mass can increase basal metabolic rate (BMR), which is the number of calories your body needs to perform basic life-sustaining functions. **Glucose Regulation:** Muscles use glucose for energy and play a significant role in maintaining normal blood sugar levels, which is important for overall metabolic health.

Roles in Metabolism Metabolism refers to all the chemical processes that occur within a living organism to maintain life. These processes include those that break down nutrients to produce energy and those that build up body structures. Here's how body fat and muscle mass influence metabolism:

Metabolic Rate: Muscle mass is more metabolically active than fat mass, meaning that individuals with higher muscle mass have a higher basal metabolic rate (BMR). This can make it easier to maintain or lose weight. **Insulin Sensitivity:** Increased muscle mass can improve insulin sensitivity, which means the body is more efficient at using glucose for energy. This reduces the risk of insulin resistance, a precursor to type 2 diabetes. **Energy Balance:** Body fat serves as an energy reserve. During periods of calorie deficit, the body can break down fat stores for energy. However, excessive body fat, especially visceral fat around the abdomen, is associated with increased risks of metabolic syndrome, type 2 diabetes, and cardiovascular diseases. Balancing body fat and muscle mass through diet and exercise is key to metabolic health. Regular physical activity, including both aerobic and resistance training, can help reduce body fat and increase or maintain muscle mass. A balanced diet rich in nutrients supports these processes by providing the necessary energy and building blocks for muscle growth and repair, while also managing calorie intake to maintain healthy body fat levels. Attaining a healthy and robust body necessitates a fundamental understanding of the key constituents that shape it. Body fat and muscle mass are crucial elements that not only influence physical appearance but also impact overall health and functionality. A comprehensive comprehension of these concepts is imperative to embark on your fitness journey with confidence and clarity. Let's demystify these concepts together and equip you with scientific knowledge to help you achieve your fitness goals.

Body fat, often vilified, is actually indispensable. It cushions our organs, insulates our bodies, and stores energy. Without it, surviving lean times would be impossible. However, like all good things, balance is key. Excessive body fat, especially visceral fat, is associated with numerous health risks, including cardiovascular disease and diabetes. On the other hand, muscle mass is the engine of your body's metabolism, burning calories even at rest. It's your ally in the battle against fat, and the more you have, the more potent your metabolic rate becomes. This doesn't just happen in the gym; it's a 24/7 process.

Understanding metabolism lays the groundwork for comprehending how body composition can be optimised. Metabolism comprises all the biochemical processes that sustain life, from converting food into energy to repairing cells. Muscle, being metabolically active, is indispensable for a healthy metabolism. Thus, the balance between muscle and fat isn't just about aesthetics; it's about health and functionality. Contrary to popular belief, simply losing weight isn't beneficial if it means losing muscle mass alongside fat.

This leads us to an essential revelation: not all weight loss is created equal. Achieving a 'fit' physique isn't solely about reducing numbers on the scale; it's about enhancing muscle mass while shedding fat. A pound of muscle is denser and occupies less space than a pound of fat, so two individuals may weigh the same but look drastically different based on their body composition. Thus, the quality of weight lost (or gained) is paramount.

How do we tilt the balance in favour of muscle mass, then? Nutrition plays a starring role. Consuming sufficient protein is vital for muscle repair and growth, while adequate caloric intake fuels both workouts and recovery. However, indiscriminate caloric surplus can lead back to fat gain, highlighting the importance of mindful eating.

Strength training emerges as a hero in this narrative. It not only builds muscle but also increases metabolic rate, contributing to greater fat loss even during rest. Imagine your body as a furnace; strength training stokes the flames, increasing the amount of fuel burned round the clock. This doesn't mean cardio is the villain. When balanced with strength training, cardio can effectively enhance fat loss without compromising muscle mass.

Transforming your body composition requires a tailored approach that considers your metabolism, lifestyle, and goals. Patience and consistency are key. Progress may be slow, but every small decision counts towards your transformation. The transformation of body composition is a combination of science and art. With the right balance of nutrition and exercise, and a good understanding and patience, you can shape your body to radiate strength, health, and vitality. This knowledge can help you in your efforts to achieve your goals.

As you progress through this book, keep in mind the relationship between body fat, muscle mass, and metabolism. Understanding this connection will help you better navigate the journey towards achieving an optimal body composition. This is not just for aesthetic reasons but also for robust health and vitality. Armed with this knowledge, coupled with determination and the right strategies, you can transform not just your body, but your entire life.

Are you interested in improving your physical fitness and exploring the intricacies of the human body? By arming ourselves with the latest scientific knowledge and a steadfast resolve, we can sculpt a resilient and vibrant physique that is a testament to our strength, dedication, and spirit. We will delve into the nuances of exercise, nutrition, and lifestyle habits, and discover the importance of discipline, consistency, and goal-setting as we work towards building a better body.

Common Misconceptions About Fat Loss and Muscle Gain

When it comes to fat loss and muscle gain, numerous misconceptions can mislead individuals about the best ways to achieve their fitness and health goals. Understanding these common myths can help set realistic expectations and foster healthier strategies for body composition changes. Here are some of the most prevalent misconceptions:

1. Spot Reduction of Fat is Possible One of the biggest myths is the idea that you can target fat loss in specific areas of the body, such as the belly, thighs, or arms, through exercises that focus on those areas. However, fat loss occurs throughout the body based on genetics, hormonal factors, and overall energy deficit, not from targeting specific muscles through exercise.

2. You Can Gain Muscle and Lose Fat Simultaneously Easily While it's not impossible, especially for beginners or those returning to exercise after a break, simultaneously gaining significant muscle while losing fat is challenging for most people. This process, often referred to as "body recomposition," requires a very balanced approach to diet and exercise, focusing on a slight calorie deficit, high protein intake, and a well-structured resistance training program.

3. High-Intensity Cardio is the Best for Fat Loss While high-intensity interval training (HIIT) can be effective for burning calories and improving cardiovascular fitness, it's not the only or necessarily the best method for fat loss for everyone. Consistency and a calorie deficit over time are more important factors. For some, moderate-intensity steady-state cardio (MISS) might be more sustainable and less taxing on the body.

4. More Protein Always Means More Muscle Protein is essential for muscle repair and growth, but there is a limit to how much muscle protein synthesis can occur at any given time. Consuming protein significantly above your body's needs will not necessarily result in more muscle gain and could potentially lead to excess calorie intake and fat gain.

5. Lifting Heavy Weights Will Make You Bulky This misconception often concerns women, who may avoid lifting heavy weights for fear of becoming too muscular. Gaining significant muscle mass requires a lot of work, a calorie surplus, and, for many, specific genetics. Resistance training, even with heavier weights, will generally result in a toned and lean physique, not bulkiness, especially under a calorie-controlled diet.

6. Supplements Are Necessary for Muscle Gain While some supplements may support muscle growth and recovery, they are not essential for everyone. A well-balanced diet rich in natural, nutrient-dense foods can meet most individuals' needs for muscle gain and maintenance. Creatine and protein supplements can be beneficial but are not necessary for everyone.

7. Eating at Night Leads to Fat Gain The timing of your meals is less important than the overall caloric balance and nutrient composition of your diet. What matters most is the total calorie intake versus expenditure over time, not necessarily when you consume those calories.

By understanding and moving past these misconceptions, individuals can adopt more effective and sustainable approaches to fat loss and muscle gain, focusing on balanced nutrition, consistent exercise, and realistic goals.

Navigating the journey towards transforming your body can often feel like trying to cut through a jungle of misinformation.

Misconceptions about fat loss and muscle gain are rampant, leading many to follow paths that may not lead to their desired destination. Understanding the truth behind these myths is crucial for setting realistic goals and adopting effective strategies.

Another widely held belief is that cutting out all fats from your diet is key to losing fat. However, dietary fats play an essential role in hormone production, including those involved in muscle growth and recovery. The key is to focus on healthy fats, such as those found in avocados, nuts, and fish, rather than eliminating fats altogether.

Similarly, the idea that carbs are the enemy is another myth that needs debunking. Carbohydrates are the body's primary energy source, especially during high-intensity workouts. Instead of cutting carbs, attention should be paid to the type and timing of carbs consumed to support your fitness goals effectively.

Many also mistakenly believe that endless hours of cardio are necessary for fat loss. While cardiovascular exercise is an important component of a well-rounded fitness plan, it's not the only, or even the most effective, way to lose fat. Strength training is equally important, as it builds muscle, which in turn can increase your resting metabolic rate, thus accelerating fat loss.

Lastly, many people think that as long as they exercise, they don't have to worry about what they eat. This couldn't be further from the truth. Nutrition plays a critical role in fat loss and muscle gain. Without paying attention to what you eat, it's difficult to achieve and maintain your body composition goals.

Clearing up these misconceptions is the first step towards adopting a more informed and effective approach to fitness. Remember, body recomposition is a journey that requires consistency, patience, and a willingness to learn and adapt. By grounding your efforts in science and realism, you can set the stage for lasting success.

The Importance of Maintaining Muscle Mass During Fat Loss

Maintaining muscle mass during fat loss is crucial for several reasons, significantly impacting your overall health, metabolic rate, and the sustainability of your fat loss efforts. Here's why it's so important:

1. Preserves Metabolic Rate Muscle tissue is metabolically active, meaning it burns calories even when you're at rest. Losing muscle mass can decrease your basal metabolic rate (BMR), which is the number of calories your body needs to perform basic functions like breathing and circulation. A higher muscle mass helps maintain a healthier metabolism, making it easier to lose fat and keep it off.

2. Improves Body Composition Body composition refers to the ratio of fat to lean mass, including muscles, bones, and organs. Aiming for fat loss while preserving muscle mass leads to a more toned and athletic appearance. This is often more desirable than simply losing weight, which can result from losing both fat and muscle.

3. Enhances Physical Strength and Functionality Muscle strength is vital for daily activities, balance, and overall physical functionality, especially as you age. Maintaining muscle mass during fat loss ensures that you not only look better but also retain (or even improve) your physical capabilities, which contributes to a better quality of life.

4. Reduces Risk of Chronic Diseases Higher muscle mass has been associated with a reduced risk of insulin resistance, type 2 diabetes, and cardiovascular disease. Muscles play a key role in glucose metabolism, helping to regulate blood sugar levels. By maintaining muscle mass, you support your body's ability to process sugars more effectively, which can lead to improved metabolic health.

5. Supports Healthy Aging As you age, you naturally lose muscle mass, a condition known as sarcopenia. This loss can lead to increased frailty and a higher risk of falls and fractures. Engaging in resistance training and ensuring adequate protein intake during weight loss can help counteract these effects, promoting healthier aging.

Strategies to Maintain Muscle Mass During Fat Loss To preserve muscle mass while losing fat, consider the following strategies:

Protein Intake: Ensure you're consuming enough protein from a variety of sources. Protein is essential for muscle repair and growth, and it also helps you feel fuller longer. **Strength Training:** Incorporate resistance or strength training into your exercise routine. This type of exercise is critical for building and maintaining muscle mass. **Caloric Deficit:** Aim for a moderate caloric deficit. Losing weight too quickly can lead to significant muscle loss alongside fat loss. **Recovery:** Allow adequate time for recovery and rest, as muscles grow and repair during rest periods. **Nutrient Timing:** Consider the timing of your nutrient intake, such as consuming a protein-rich meal or snack after a workout to support muscle repair. By focusing on maintaining muscle mass during fat loss, you can achieve a healthier, more sustainable transformation that benefits your appearance, strength, and overall health.

Maintaining muscle mass during a fat loss journey is essential for achieving long-term success and sustainability of your results. It requires a nuanced understanding of body composition and a commitment to balance in your diet and exercise regimen. The goal is to lose fat while preserving muscle mass, which involves more than just reducing calorie intake or increasing physical activity. You need to fine-tune your approach to exercise and nutrition to ensure that your body doesn't break down muscle tissue for energy. This is a strategic endeavor that requires a thoughtful and balanced approach.

Why is muscle mass so crucial, you ask? For starters, muscle tissue is metabolically active as previously mentioned, meaning it burns calories even when you're not moving. This is a stark contrast to fat tissue, which has a much lower metabolic rate. In essence, the more muscle mass you have, the higher your resting metabolic rate (RMR) will be. This doesn't just have implications for weight loss but for your overall health and vitality. A higher RMR means your body is burning more calories at rest, making it easier to maintain a healthy weight or lose fat when that's your goal.

During a calorie deficit, the body is forced to find alternative energy sources to compensate for the lack of incoming energy from food. Ideally, it would turn to its fat stores, but without the right balance of nutrients and exercise, muscle can also become a target. This is why just cutting calories isn't enough. Protein intake, for example, needs to be adequate to protect and repair muscle tissue. Not to mention, engaging in strength training sends a signal to your body that muscle needs to be preserved for these demanding tasks.

Strength training is a cornerstone in the quest to maintain muscle mass. It not only helps build muscle but also aids in preserving it when you're in a calorie deficit. It does this by promoting muscle protein synthesis, essentially telling your body that the muscle is still needed and shouldn't be broken down for energy. This kind of training comes in various forms, from traditional weight lifting to bodyweight exercises, allowing a range of options depending on what's available to you or your personal preferences.

Another important aspect is the role of dietary protein. It cannot be overstated how instrumental protein is in the muscle maintenance process. Adequate protein intake supports muscle synthesis and repair, especially important during periods of calorie restriction. This means not just hitting a minimum protein target but also distributing protein intake evenly throughout the day to maximise muscle protein synthesis.

Beyond the biochemical and physiological considerations, there's a psychological component to retaining muscle mass. Seeing your strength improve and your physique become more defined can be incredibly motivating. It's a tangible sign that your efforts are paying off, underscoring the importance of pairing fat loss goals with strength and muscle maintenance for both physical and mental rewards.

However, balance is key. It's possible to overdo it, either with excessive calorie restriction or overtraining, both of which can lead to muscle loss. Listening to your body is crucial. Rest and recovery are just as important as your diet and training regimen. They allow your muscles to repair and grow stronger, readying them for the next challenge. This strategic approach ensures that you're losing fat, not muscle.

To sum up, maintaining muscle mass during fat loss is a multifaceted endeavour that hinges on a balanced diet rich in protein, a carefully crafted exercise regimen that includes strength training, and adequate rest. By paying close attention to these elements, you can ensure that your fat loss journey leads to a stronger, leaner, and more resilient body. This is not just about aesthetics but about fostering good health and a higher quality of life for years to come.

Chapter 2:
The Science of Fat Loss and Muscle Gain

It is worth noting that building muscle and losing fat at the same time may not be the most efficient way to achieve your desired physique. For some individuals, it may be more effective to focus on building muscle first and then transitioning to a fat loss phase. This depends on where you start out, some might need to lose fat first.

When you focus on building muscle, you need to consume more calories than your body needs to support muscle growth. This will inevitably lead to some fat gain, but the overall result will be an increase in muscle mass. Once you have built a solid foundation of muscle, you can then transition to a fat loss phase where you will consume fewer calories to shed the excess fat.

This approach allows you to focus on one goal at a time, which can be more effective than trying to achieve two conflicting goals simultaneously. It also allows you to build a solid foundation of muscle, which will help support your fat loss efforts by increasing your metabolism and making it easier to maintain your weight.

In summary, while it is possible to lose fat and gain muscle simultaneously, it may not be the most efficient approach for everyone. Depending on your goals and individual circumstances, it may be more effective to focus on building muscle first and then transitioning to a fat loss phase. Again remember that some might need to start by loosing fat first.

Hormones also play in important role in our bodycomposition. Hormones such as testosterone and growth hormone play a major role in muscle synthesis. On the other hand, insulin and cortisol influence fat storage and utilization. Therefore, understanding how to optimize these hormones naturally through proper nutrition, resistance training, and lifestyle changes can be a powerful tool in achieving our fitness goals.

Additionally, comprehending the concept of energy balance, which is the balance between calories consumed and calories burned, provides a clear and flexible framework for achieving a leaner, more muscular physique over time. This chapter focuses on providing you with the scientific principles needed to navigate your fitness journey and emphasizes that with knowledge, dedication, and a strategic approach.

An Overview of How the Body Loses Fat and Builds Muscle

Losing fat and gaining muscle is a complex process that depends on metabolism, hormones, and recovery. This overview will explain how the body burns fat, builds muscle, and why recovery is crucial.

Understanding Fat Loss The Principle of Caloric Deficit At the heart of fat loss lies the principle of energy balance: consuming fewer calories than the body expends leads to a caloric deficit, compelling the body to tap into stored fat for energy. This metabolic shift triggers fat breakdown, known as lipolysis, where triglycerides are converted into glycerol and free fatty acids for fuel.

Hormonal Influence on Fat Metabolism Hormones such as insulin, cortisol, and the duo of leptin and ghrelin orchestrate appetite, fat storage, and energy utilization. Insulin's role in glucose regulation affects fat storage, whereas cortisol can promote fat accumulation under chronic stress. Leptin and ghrelin, the satiety and hunger hormones respectively, modulate appetite and can influence body weight.

The Pathway to Muscle Growth The Mechanics of Muscle Hypertrophy Muscle growth, or hypertrophy, is spurred by resistance training that induces micro-damage to muscle fibers. This physical stress, coupled with adequate nutritional support, particularly protein, initiates repair processes that thicken and strengthen muscle fibers, contributing to muscle volume and strength.

Nutritional Building Blocks Adequate protein intake is crucial for muscle repair and growth. Amino acids from protein serve as the building blocks for new muscle tissue, underscoring the importance of protein-rich foods and supplements in the diet of anyone looking to gain muscle.

Role of Hormones in Muscle Development Testosterone and growth hormone significantly impact muscle synthesis and repair. These hormones increase protein synthesis, muscle mass, and strength, highlighting the importance of not only training and nutrition but also optimal hormonal balance for muscle growth.

The Crucial Role of Recovery Rest and Muscle Repair Recovery is not merely a passive phase but an active component of fitness where the body repairs, rebuilds, and strengthens tissues. Adequate rest, including sleep and days off from intense training, allows for muscular repair and growth, underscoring the need for well-planned rest days in any training regimen.

Nutrition and Hydration for Recovery Post-workout nutrition is pivotal in kickstarting the recovery process. Consuming carbohydrates and protein soon after exercise replenishes energy stores and accelerates muscle repair. Hydration is equally important, as water supports metabolic functions and nutrient transfer within the body.

The Indispensable Need for Sleep Sleep is the pinnacle of recovery. During sleep, the body undergoes profound healing, growth hormone levels surge, and muscle repair is optimized. Inadequate sleep can disrupt hormonal balance, impair recovery, and even lead to gains in fat mass over time.

In summary, the processes of losing fat and building muscle are interlinked, requiring a meticulous approach to diet, exercise, and, recovery. Understanding these processes allows for a more informed and effective approach to fitness, emphasizing the body's complex response to exercise, nutrition, and rest.

The Role of Hormones in Fat Loss and Muscle Growth

Our body is a complex system that relies on a multitude of factors to maintain proper function. Hormones play a crucial role in regulating these functions and are often referred to as the "messengers" of the body. Hormones travel through our bloodstream and interact with specific cells to influence various processes, including fat loss and muscle growth.

Insulin: First and foremost, let's talk about insulin. Often villainised in the world of dieting, insulin is actually indispensable for muscle growth. It promotes the uptake of glucose into cells, fuelling our workouts and aiding in the recovery and growth of muscle tissue. However, maintaining a balance is key. Excessive insulin spikes, often a result of a high-sugar diet, can lead to increased fat storage. Thus, managing insulin levels through a well-balanced diet is a cornerstone of body recomposition. There are times when you do want a sugary spike to release more insuling, this is during and after a training session to aid recovery.

Consuming high-glycemic carbohydrates (like dextrose) during or after your workout induces an insulin spike. The insulin spike enhances the uptake of these nutrients by muscle cells, which can be beneficial for recovery and growth. This is particularly important post-workout when your muscles are in a state primed for nutrient absorption.

Exercise depletes muscle glycogen stores, and consuming fast-acting carbohydrates helps replenish these stores more quickly. Glycogen is the primary fuel source for high-intensity exercise, and its replenishment is crucial for recovery and performance in subsequent workouts. By providing a quick source of energy and supporting insulin-mediated pathways, these sugars can help minimize muscle breakdown and promote repair processes.

Insulin is not just a nutrient transporter but also an anabolic hormone. By spiking insulin levels at the right time, it can help create a more favorable environment for muscle growth. The combination of insulin with amino acids (either from protein consumed simultaneously or circulating in the bloodstream) can stimulate muscle protein synthesis, a key process in muscle repair and growth.

Supplements that act like insulin or promote insulin sensitivity can play a role in managing blood sugar levels, especially for individuals with diabetes or those at risk of developing diabetes. However, it's crucial to consult with a healthcare provider before starting any new supplement, especially for those with existing health conditions or those taking medication. Here are some supplements known to influence insulin sensitivity:

Alpha-lipoic acid (ALA): ALA is an antioxidant that has been shown to improve insulin sensitivity and reduce symptoms of diabetic neuropathy. It helps cells absorb glucose more effectively. **Chromium:** Chromium is a trace mineral that enhances the action of insulin and is involved in carbohydrate, fat, and protein metabolism. Some studies suggest that chromium supplementation may improve insulin sensitivity and glucose metabolism. **Magnesium:** Low levels of magnesium are linked to insulin resistance. Supplementing with magnesium may improve insulin sensitivity in individuals with a deficiency. **Berberine:** This compound, found in several plants, is shown to significantly reduce blood sugar levels in individuals with type 2 diabetes, potentially by improving insulin sensitivity and enhancing glucose uptake by the cells. **Cinnamon:** Cinnamon may improve insulin sensitivity by increasing glucose uptake into cells. Some studies suggest it can mimic insulin and act on insulin receptors. **Omega-3 fatty acids:** Found in fish oil and flaxseed, omega-3s can improve insulin sensitivity and reduce inflammation. Green tea extract: Epigallocatechin gallate (EGCG), a component of green tea, may enhance insulin sensitivity. **Vitamin D:** Vitamin D deficiency is linked to increased risk of insulin resistance. Correcting a deficiency may improve insulin sensitivity. **Resveratrol:** Found in the skin of red grapes, resveratrol has been shown to improve insulin sensitivity and mimic the effects of calorie restriction. **Bitter melon:** Contains compounds that act like insulin, helping to lower blood sugar levels and increase cellular uptake of glucose. **Gymnema Sylvestre:** Referred to as the "sugar destroyer," it may help reduce sugar cravings and improve glucose control.

These supplements can interact with medications and may not be suitable for everyone. It's essential to approach the use of supplements cautiously and under the guidance of a healthcare provider to ensure they are used safely and effectively.

Testosterone: Testosterone and growth hormone (GH) are the superheroes when it comes to muscle building and fat loss. Testosterone facilitates muscle growth by stimulating protein synthesis and inhibiting protein breakdown, making it a critical factor for gaining strength and size.

Testosterone plays a crucial role in muscle building and fat loss, significantly impacting body composition and overall physical performance. Here's a breakdown of how testosterone influences these processes:

Testosterone increases the rate of protein synthesis in the body. Muscle growth occurs when the rate of protein synthesis exceeds the rate of protein breakdown. Higher levels of testosterone accelerate protein synthesis, leading to muscle hypertrophy (growth). After a workout, muscles need to repair and rebuild through a process that requires protein. Testosterone helps increase the body's ability to rebuild and repair muscle tissues, speeding up recovery times and making muscles stronger and larger as a response to exercise. Testosterone can decrease the activity of catabolic hormones in the body, which are responsible for breaking down muscle tissue. By reducing the effects of these hormones, testosterone helps preserve muscle mass, making it easier to build and maintain muscle.

Supplements to Increase Testosterone:

Vitamin D: Often referred to as a hormone, Vitamin D is crucial for maintaining healthy levels of testosterone. Supplementation can be particularly beneficial for individuals with low sunlight exposure or Vitamin D deficiency.

D-Aspartic Acid: An amino acid that has been shown to potentially boost testosterone levels by increasing the release of a hormone in the brain that ultimately results in testosterone production. However, results can vary, and more research is needed to confirm its efficacy.

Fenugreek: An herb that has been linked to increased testosterone levels and improved libido. Fenugreek may also enhance muscle strength and fat loss when combined with resistance training.

Zinc: An essential mineral involved in over 100 chemical processes in the body, including testosterone production. Zinc supplementation has been shown to increase testosterone levels, especially in men with low zinc status.

Ashwagandha: This adaptogen has been studied for its ability to increase testosterone levels, particularly in men with stress-related fertility issues. It may also improve exercise performance, strength, and fat loss.

Estrogen: Estrogen significantly influences fat loss and muscle gain in both men and women, albeit in different ways, affecting body composition, metabolism, and the distribution of body fat.

Estrogen determines fat storage locations: in women, typically in the hips, buttocks, and thighs; in men, around the abdomen. Metabolic Rate: It subtly affects the basal metabolic rate (BMR), interacting with hormones that regulate metabolism and impacting weight management. Estrogen fluctuations can influence hunger and satiety hormones, affecting eating behaviors and ultimately body weight. It plays a role in muscle tissue repair post-exercise by modulating inflammatory responses and enhancing muscle growth through the activation of satellite cells. Estrogen contributes to muscle strength and function, with its receptors found in muscle tissues influencing metabolism and contractile properties. Offers antioxidant properties that protect muscles from exercise-induced oxidative stress, aiding in recovery and performance.

Gender Differences Women's higher estrogen levels lead to a higher body fat percentage and efficient fat storage, a trait linked to fertility. Men, with lower estrogen and higher testosterone, tend to have a leaner mass with more muscle. However, balanced estrogen levels are crucial for both genders for optimal health, affecting fat distribution, muscle growth, and metabolic health.

Managing estrogen levels can be important for both men and women, especially for those experiencing hormonal imbalances that affect their health and body composition. Several supplements are purported to help regulate or manage estrogen levels.

Supplements to help balance estrogen.

Diindolylmethane (DIM) DIM is a compound found naturally in cruciferous vegetables like broccoli, Brussels sprouts, and cabbage. It's believed to support the metabolism of estrogen, converting it to less potent forms. This can potentially aid in balancing estrogen levels and is often used by individuals looking to manage estrogen dominance.

Calcium-D-Glucarate This substance is thought to help detoxify and remove excess estrogen from the body. It does so by inhibiting the enzyme beta-glucuronidase, thereby promoting the excretion of estrogen through the digestive tract. Calcium-D-Glucarate is found in fruits and vegetables, such as oranges, apples, and grapefruit.

Indole-3-Carbinol (I3C) I3C is another compound found in cruciferous vegetables. In the body, it's converted to DIM, offering similar potential benefits in estrogen metabolism. I3C is thought to promote the conversion of estrogen to less potent forms, which might help in maintaining a healthier estrogen balance.

Chrysin Chrysin is a flavonoid found in honey, propolis, and some plants. It's often marketed as a supplement to boost testosterone and reduce estrogen levels. However, its effectiveness in reducing estrogen when taken orally is debated, as its bioavailability is relatively low.

Resveratrol Resveratrol is a polyphenolic compound found in red wine, grapes, and berries. It has been studied for various health benefits, including its potential to act as an estrogen antagonist. By modulating estrogen receptors and metabolism, resveratrol might help in maintaining estrogen balance.

Zinc Zinc is an essential mineral that plays a role in hormone balance, including testosterone and estrogen. It's thought to inhibit the enzyme aromatase, which converts testosterone to estrogen. Adequate zinc levels can help maintain hormonal balance and support overall reproductive health.

Growth Hormone: (GH), also known as somatotropin, is a peptide hormone that plays a vital role in growth, body composition, cell repair, and metabolism. GH influences muscle building and fat loss in several significant ways, making it crucial for physical development and maintenance.GH directly stimulates the growth of muscle tissues partly by promoting cell division and multiplication even if this is not often seen to an extent where one would notice it. It can though increase the number of muscle cells (hyperplasia) and can enhance muscle cell size (hypertrophy) through its effects on protein synthesis. Similar to testosterone, GH increases the rate of protein synthesis in skeletal muscle. It enhances the uptake of amino acids into muscle cells, providing the necessary building blocks for muscle growth and repair, which is essential after rigorous exercise.

GH plays a critical role in the repair and recovery of muscle tissues damaged during workouts. It stimulates the regeneration of tissue, helps to repair muscle fibers, and reduces recovery time, allowing for more frequent and intensive training sessions. Increases Insulin-like Growth Factor 1 (IGF-1) Production: GH stimulates the liver to produce IGF-1, a hormone that has powerful anabolic effects in the body. IGF-1 is crucial for muscle growth as it enhances both the differentiation and proliferation of myoblasts (muscle cells), leading to increased muscle mass and strength.

Supplements to Increase Growth Hormone (GH)

Arginine: taken alone, without exercise, arginine may boost GH levels. It's often taken in high doses by those looking to enhance their GH profile for fitness and recovery purposes.

Gamma-Aminobutyric Acid: (GABA)A neurotransmitter that can help to increase GH levels when taken before sleep or exercise. GABA is also known for its calming effects on the brain.

Melatonin: Known primarily for its role in regulating sleep cycles, melatonin supplementation can also increase GH levels, as GH secretion is naturally higher during sleep.

Beta-Alanine: Often used to enhance exercise performance, beta-alanine has been shown to increase exercise-induced GH levels, particularly in response to intense resistance training.

L-Glutamine: A small amount of evidence suggests that short-term supplementation of high doses of glutamine may promote an increase in GH levels. However, more research is needed to fully understand its effects.

Cortisol: Next on the list is cortisol, known as the stress hormone. While it plays a necessary role in functions like controlling blood sugar levels and regulating metabolism, chronic high levels of cortisol can lead to muscle breakdown and increased abdominal fat. Thus, strategies for managing stress and ensuring adequate sleep become indispensable parts of a fitness regimen focused on muscle growth and fat loss.

Leptin and ghrelin, the hunger hormones, also play significant roles in fat loss. Leptin signals satiety, helping to regulate energy balance and reduce food intake, whereas ghrelin stimulates appetite. Fluctuations in these hormones can challenge one's adherence to a diet. Yet, by focusing on a diet rich in fibre, protein, and healthy fats, we can modulate these hormonal signals to support our fat loss goals.

Thyroid hormones, T3 (Triiodothyronine) and T4 (Thyroxine) are hormones produced by the thyroid gland, which plays a crucial role in regulating metabolism, energy production, and overall physical and mental development. The balance of these hormones is essential for maintaining optimal health, as well as for fat loss and muscle gain. Here's a breakdown of their roles from a health, fat loss, and muscle gain perspective:

Health Perspective T3 and T4 Regulation: These hormones help regulate the body's metabolic rate, influencing how fast or slow your body uses energy. Proper levels are essential for the normal functioning of various systems in the body, including the heart, muscles, and digestive system. Energy and Mood: Adequate levels of T3 and T4 contribute to normal energy levels and mood. Imbalances can lead to conditions such as hypothyroidism (low hormone levels) or hyperthyroidism (high hormone levels), affecting overall well-being and mental health.

Fat Loss Perspective Metabolic Rate: T3, the more active form of thyroid hormone, significantly impacts your metabolic rate. Higher levels of T3 can increase energy expenditure, helping with fat loss. However, excessively high levels can be detrimental and should not be targeted through unsupervised supplementation. Appetite and Energy Use: Normal levels of thyroid hormones help in maintaining a balanced appetite and efficient use of dietary energy. Disruptions can lead to weight gain or difficulty losing weight.

Muscle Gain Perspective Protein Synthesis: Thyroid hormones are involved in protein synthesis, which is crucial for muscle repair and growth. Adequate levels support the building of muscle mass. Metabolic Support: By supporting a healthy metabolic rate, T3 and T4 can aid in creating an environment conducive to muscle gain, provided that diet and exercise are appropriately managed.

Maintaining Healthy Levels Maintaining healthy levels of T3 and T4 usually involves managing your overall health and thyroid function. While specific supplements can support thyroid health, it's crucial to approach this under medical supervision, as improper use can lead to health issues. Here are some general tips:

Iodine: This mineral is critical for thyroid hormone production. Foods rich in iodine include seaweed, fish, dairy, and eggs. Iodine supplements should be taken cautiously, as both too little and too much can disrupt thyroid function. Selenium: Selenium helps in the conversion of T4 to T3. Brazil nuts, seafood, and meats are good sources. **Zinc:** Zinc also supports the conversion of T4 to T3. Foods like oysters, beef, and pumpkin seeds are rich in zinc.

Ashwagandha: this may help in regulating the synthesis of thyroid hormones. It has been shown in some studies to stimulate the production of thyroid hormones, particularly T4 (thyroxine). This can be particularly beneficial for individuals with hypothyroidism, where the thyroid gland is underactive and produces insufficient amounts of thyroid hormones. Ashwagandha is known for its adaptogenic properties, meaning it helps the body adapt to stress. By mitigating stress and reducing cortisol levels, ashwagandha can indirectly support thyroid function. High cortisol levels can interfere with thyroid hormone production and balance, so managing stress is crucial for maintaining healthy thyroid function.

Important Considerations Individual Responses: The effectiveness of these supplements can vary widely among individuals. Factors such as age, baseline hormone levels, lifestyle, and overall health status can influence results. Medical Supervision: Before starting any supplement regimen to increase hormone levels, consult with a healthcare provider. They can offer guidance based on your specific health needs and conditions and monitor your hormone levels. **Holistic Approach:** Supplements may offer support, but a holistic approach that includes a balanced diet, regular exercise, adequate sleep, and stress management is crucial for optimizing hormone levels and overall health. **Quality and Safety:** Choose high-quality supplements from reputable manufacturers to avoid contaminants and ensure the product contains what it claims.

Increasing testosterone and GH levels naturally involves a multifaceted approach. While supplements can play a role, they should be part of a broader lifestyle strategy aimed at enhancing overall health and hormonal balance.

It's clear that hormones are integral in determining how our bodies respond to diet and exercise. However, it's also evident that we can influence these hormonal responses through our lifestyle choices. By focusing on resistance training, managing stress, optimising sleep, and adhering to a balanced diet, we can create an internal environment conducive to fat loss and muscle growth.

To sum it up, recognising the role of hormones in shaping our physique opens up a new dimension of strategy in fitness. It transitions us from a simplistic calorie-in-calorie-out approach to a more nuanced understanding of body recomposition. This knowledge empowers us to fine-tune our diet and exercise plans, paving the way for more efficient and sustainable results.

By understanding the role that hormones play in fat loss and muscle growth, we can better tailor our diet and exercise routines to achieve our desired body composition. For example, eating a diet that regulates insulin levels, such as a low-carbohydrate diet, can help promote fat loss. Additionally, engaging in regular strength training exercises can help increase both testosterone and GH levels and promote muscle growth.

The Concept of Energy Balance and Its Implications for Body Recomposition

The concept of energy balance is fundamental to understanding how the body gains, loses, or maintains weight, which is crucial for anyone looking to undergo body recomposition. Body recomposition refers to the process of changing one's physique by reducing body fat and increasing muscle mass simultaneously or in a phased approach.

Understanding Energy Balance Energy balance is the relationship between the energy (calories) you take in through food and drink and the energy your body uses for things like basic functioning (basal metabolic rate or BMR), physical activity, and processing food (thermic effect of food).

Caloric Surplus: When you consume more calories than your body needs, you're in a caloric surplus. The body stores the excess energy as fat, leading to weight gain. **Caloric Deficit:** When you consume fewer calories than your body uses, you're in a caloric deficit. The body then turns to stored fat (and sometimes muscle) for energy, leading to weight loss. **Energy Balance:** When the calories consumed match the calories used, you're in energy balance, maintaining your current weight.

Implications for Body Recomposition Body recomposition is about tweaking this energy balance to support fat loss while either maintaining or gaining muscle mass. This can be challenging because the traditional approach to losing weight (being in a caloric deficit) can also lead to muscle loss, while gaining muscle typically requires a caloric surplus. Here's how the concept of energy balance can be applied to body recomposition:

Moderate Caloric Deficit: A slight caloric deficit can encourage fat loss while minimizing the risk of muscle loss, especially if protein intake is high and resistance training is part of your routine. **Increased**

Protein Intake: Protein supports muscle repair and growth. Consuming enough protein can help preserve muscle mass during a calorie deficit and is essential for building muscle. **Resistance Training:** Engaging in resistance training stimulates muscle growth, which can occur even in a caloric deficit if the deficit is not too severe and nutrition is optimized. This training is crucial for adding or maintaining muscle mass while losing fat. **Nutrient Timing and Quality:** Focusing on the quality of your diet and the timing of nutrient intake (e.g., consuming protein and carbs after a workout) can also support muscle synthesis and recovery while in a deficit. **Recomposition Phases:** Some individuals may find it easier to focus on either fat loss or muscle gain in separate phases while maintaining the other. This phased approach can make managing the energy balance and dietary requirements more straightforward.

Long-Term Considerations Body recomposition is generally a slower process than traditional weight loss or muscle-building strategies. It requires patience, persistence, and a nuanced approach to diet and exercise. Adjustments to your plan may be necessary as your body changes and adapts.

Understanding and applying the principles of energy balance in the context of your lifestyle, goals, and body's responses is critical. It's not just about calories in versus calories out; it's about the quality of those calories, the timing, and how they support your specific training and recovery needs. Transforming one's body by losing fat and gaining muscle is a difficult task. Energy balance is a crucial concept at the heart of this process and cannot be overlooked. It is a fundamental principle that plays a vital role in achieving the desired results.

At its core, the principle of energy balance sounds straightforward – consume more calories than you expend to gain weight, and consume fewer to lose weight. However, when delving into body recomposition, the goal isn't just about shifting numbers on a scale; it's about strategically losing fat while gaining or preserving muscle mass. This nuanced approach necessitates a more sophisticated understanding of how different macronutrients and exercise regimes influence energy expenditure and muscle synthesis.

Fat loss and muscle gain are strictly physiological processes that are governed by the body's hormonal landscape, which, in turn, is solely influenced by one's diet and exercise routines. Hormones like insulin, testosterone, growth hormone and glucagon play critical roles in these processes, but it's the energy balance that is the most important.

To achieve body recomposition, one must be extremely disciplined and maintain a slight caloric deficit or balancing just on the edge of your maintenance level to trigger fat loss while also ensuring adequate protein intake and engaging in rigorous resistance training to stimulate muscle growth. This delicate balance between calories and nutritional sufficiency is what makes the concept of energy balance both a science and an art, and it requires strict adherence to achieve desired results.

Resistance training is crucial in this equation. Not only does it contribute to an increase in muscle mass, which in turn elevates basal metabolic rate (the amount of energy expended while at rest), but it also ensures that a caloric deficit preferentially targets fat stores over muscle tissue. This dual role underscores the importance of integrating strength training into any body recomposition strategy.

Nutritional strategies play a significant role as well. A diet high in protein supports muscle synthesis and repair, while ensuring the body feels satiated, which can help prevent overeating. Understanding the roles of carbohydrates and fats is also essential, as they influence energy levels and hormonal responses, respectively, both of which are crucial for optimizing body recomposition.

Embracing the concept of energy balance doesn't mean adhering to a rigid, one-size-fits-all formula. It involves a dynamic and personalized approach that considers not only total caloric intake but also the quality and timing of those calories. This tailored approach ensures that one can effectively lose fat and build muscle without compromising health or vitality.

Chapter 3:
Nutrition for Fat Loss and Muscle Preservation

Achieving fat loss while preserving muscle mass requires a highly precise and demanding approach to nutrition. Understanding the underlying physiological mechanisms and developing a meticulously crafted strategy that aligns with an individual's body needs are crucial components of this complex task. At the core of this is the delicate manipulation of macronutrients – proteins, fats, and carbohydrates - to achieve a state of negative energy balance that promotes fat loss while preserving or even increasing muscle mass.

A high-protein diet, typically defined as the daily consumption of at least 1.6-2 grams of protein per kilogram of body weight, is not only crucial for muscle repair and growth but also plays a key role in satiety and energy expenditure, thus facilitating fat loss. However, the role of carbohydrates and fats in the context of a weight loss diet cannot be understated, as they provide the necessary fuel for physical activity and basal metabolism, ensuring that the body does not resort to muscle stores for energy. Achieving the right caloric balance is crucial, as it involves reducing calorie intake sufficiently to trigger fat loss without compromising muscle mass, a balance that hinges on precise calorie tracking and understanding the thermic effect of food, which refers to the energy expenditure required to digest, absorb, and metabolize dietary nutrients.

Timing nutrient intake to support energy needs and recovery, particularly around exercise, can further optimize the balance between fat loss and muscle preservation. Including strategic supplementation, such as essential amino acids (EAAs) or whey protein, may offer an additional edge in muscle recovery and growth, providing the body with essential amino acids at critical times with less calories than you would get from most foods as these supplements can contain almost next to no other calories from carbs or fats. Ultimately, successful nutrition for fat loss and muscle preservation requires a long-term, sustainable approach that respects individual body's requirements and preferences, and is supported by sound scientific principles.

Macronutrients: Roles, How Much You Need, and Best Sources

Achieving fat loss and muscle preservation requires a clear understanding of macronutrients, which are the essential components of nutrition that help shape the body. Proteins, carbohydrates, and fats are the three macronutrients that play distinctive roles in the composition and function of our body.

Protein Role in Muscle Gain:

Muscle Repair and Growth: Protein is essential for repairing and building muscle tissue, especially after exercise. It provides amino acids, the building blocks of muscle, which stimulate muscle protein synthesis (MPS), the process leading to increased muscle mass. Satiety and Preservation of Lean Mass: High-protein diets increase feelings of fullness, which can help reduce overall calorie intake. During weight loss, a higher protein intake can help preserve lean muscle mass, ensuring most weight loss comes from fat.

Role in Fat Loss:

Thermic Effect: Protein has a higher thermic effect compared to carbohydrates and fats, meaning your body uses more energy to digest and metabolize it. This increased energy expenditure can contribute to fat loss. Maintains Metabolism: By preserving lean muscle mass during weight loss, protein helps maintain a healthy metabolism, as muscle tissue burns more calories at rest than fat tissue.

The general recommendation for those engaging in regular strength training is to consume approximately 1.6 to 2.2 grams of protein per kilogram of body weight daily. High-quality protein can be sourced from poultry, lean meats, fish, dairy, and plant-based alternatives like lentils and chickpeas.

Carbohydrates Role in Muscle Gain:

Energy for Workouts: Carbohydrates are the body's primary energy source during high-intensity workouts. Adequate carb intake helps replenish glycogen stores in muscles, supporting endurance and performance, thereby enabling more intense training sessions that can lead to muscle gain. Supports Muscle Recovery: Consuming carbs post-workout can enhance glycogen replenishment and, when paired with protein, improve protein synthesis, aiding in muscle recovery and growth.

Role in Fat Loss:

Fuel for Exercise: While carbs are essential for fueling exercise, moderating carbohydrate intake based on your activity level can help create the calorie deficit needed for fat loss without compromising energy levels for workouts. Fiber Intake: High-fiber carbohydrates (like vegetables, whole grains, and legumes) can enhance feelings of fullness, leading to reduced calorie intake and aiding in fat loss.

Carbohydrates, often misunderstood, are your body's primary energy provider. They fuel your workouts and aid in recovery. Depending on your activity level, carbohydrates should constitute about 45% to 65% of your total caloric intake. Opt for whole sources like fruits, vegetables, whole grains, and legumes to get the most benefit and sustained energy release.

Fats Role in Muscle Gain:

Hormone Production: Fats are crucial for the production of hormones like testosterone and growth hormone, both of which are involved in muscle growth. Ensuring an adequate intake of healthy fats can support an optimal hormonal environment for muscle gain. **Energy Source:** Fats provide a concentrated source of energy, which can be particularly useful for fueling longer, lower-intensity workouts or supporting overall calorie needs for those on high-calorie diets to gain muscle.

Role in Fat Loss:

Satiety and Nutrient Absorption: Fats are digested slowly, which can help increase satiety and reduce overall calorie intake. They also aid in the absorption of fat-soluble vitamins, supporting overall health during calorie-restricted diets. **Choosing the Right Fats:** Incorporating healthy fats (such as those from avocados, nuts, seeds, and fish) instead of saturated and trans fats can support heart health and overall well-being, aligning with long-term fat loss and maintenance goals.

Fats should not be shunned in your diet; they're essential for hormone production, including those involved in muscle growth and fat loss. Dietary fats should account for 20% to 30% of your total calories, focusing on sources rich in unsaturated fats, such as avocados, nuts, seeds, and olive oil.

Understanding the balance and importance of each macronutrient is key. It's not just about hitting your daily caloric needs; it's about fuelling your body with the right proportions of macros to support fat loss while preserving muscle mass.

To put this into practice, start by calculating your daily caloric expenditure and adjust based on your specific goals. Include a variety of sources for each macronutrient to ensure you're not only meeting your macro goals but also consuming a wide range of micronutrients essential for overall health.

Calculating your daily calorie expenditure involves understanding the total amount of calories you burn in a day, which includes your basal metabolic rate (BMR), the thermic effect of food (TEF), and calories burned through physical activity. We will dive deeper into this in the next chapter.

Remember, consistency is more powerful than perfection. Small, manageable adjustments to your diet, centered around macronutrient balance, will accumulate over time leading to significant changes in your body composition.

Moreover, hydration plays a crucial role in this process. Water assists in nutrient transport and helps maintain optimal performance during workouts. Don't overlook the importance of drinking enough water throughout the day.

Finally, knowing that nutrition is not one-size-fits-all, feel empowered to tweak and adjust your macronutrient intake based on your progress and how your body responds. This journey is as much about learning what works for your body as it is about achieving your goals.

As you move forward, remember the power of nutrition in transforming your body. It's the fuel for your journey towards fat loss and muscle preservation. With the right knowledge and application of macronutrients, you're well on your way to achieving and sustaining your fitness goals.

Caloric Deficits: How to Calculate and Maintain Without Losing Muscle

Fat loss requires a nuanced approach; it's not just about shedding pounds but doing so in a way that preserves, or even enhances, muscle mass. At the heart of this process is creating and managing a caloric deficit—the fundamental principle of fat loss—without compromising muscle. The science might sound complex, but it boils down to the energy balance equation: consume fewer calories than you expend. However, the challenge here is to strike the right balance so that your body resorts to burning fat for energy, rather than breaking down muscle tissue.

To calculate your caloric deficit, you need to first understand your Total Daily Energy Expenditure (TDEE).

Here's a simple way to estimate your daily calorie expenditure:

Step 1: Calculate Your BMR BMR is the number of calories your body needs to perform basic life-sustaining functions, like breathing and circulating blood. You can estimate your BMR using the Harris-Benedict Equation, which has different calculations for men and women:

For men: BMR = 88.362 + (13.397 × weight in kg) + (4.799 × height in cm) - (5.677 × age in years) For women: BMR = 447.593 + (9.247 × weight in kg) + (3.098 × height in cm) - (4.330 × age in years)

Step 2: Account for Physical Activity Multiply your BMR by the appropriate physical activity level (PAL) to account for calories burned through movement. Here are general PAL values:

Sedentary (little or no exercise): BMR × 1.2 Lightly active (light exercise/sports 1-3 days/week): BMR × 1.375 Moderately active (moderate exercise/sports 3-5 days/week): BMR × 1.55 Very active (hard exercise/sports 6-7 days a week): BMR × 1.725 Extra active (very hard exercise/sports & a physical job): BMR × 1.9

Example Calculation: Calculate BMR (for a 30-year-old woman, 65 kg, 170 cm tall): 447.593 + (9.247 × 65) + (3.098 × 170) - (4.330 × 30) = 1,447 calories Adjust for Activity Level (moderately active): 1,447 × 1.55 = 2,243 calories

This example woman would burn approximately 2,243 calories in a day.

If you want to gain muscle and loose fat at the same start with this number (2,243 in the example) and adjust your deficit with extra cardio or daily activity like step count. If fat loss is your primary goal, start with decreasing this number by 20% and adjust on a weekly basis. Same thing if you already are fairly lean and your focus is muscle gain with minimal fat gain start by increasing your daily calorie expenditure with 15-20% and ajust thereafter. This method provides a rough estimate of your daily calorie expenditure. For a more accurate assessment, consider using a fitness tracker or consulting a health professional.

However, not all calories are equal, especially when your goal is to retain muscle mass. This is where macronutrient distribution comes into play. Proteins, in particular, are paramount for muscle preservation. Studies have shown that higher protein diets, in the context of a caloric deficit, help in retaining lean muscle mass. Carbohydrates and fats are also necessary, but their proportions can be more flexible, tailored to your lifestyle and preferences.

Maintaining muscle while in a caloric deficit isn't just about what you eat, but also about how you train. Strength training is non-negotiable here. It sends a clear signal to your body that the muscle is needed, which in turn helps to preserve it even when you're cutting calories. Aim for at least 3 full body sessions a week if you dont have the time for a more split focused approach, focusing on compound movements that recruit multiple muscle groups for maximum efficiency.

Many fear that a caloric deficit means constant hunger and deprivation, but it doesn't have to be that way. Volume eating—focusing on foods high in volume but low in calories—can help keep you full. Think vegetables, fruits, and lean proteins. Hydration is equally critical, as thirst can sometimes be misinterpreted as hunger.

Rest and recovery are also vital components of muscle preservation. When you're in a caloric deficit, your body can perceive this as stress. Without adequate sleep and rest days, cortisol levels might rise, potentially leading to muscle breakdown. Hence, ensuring quality sleep and incorporating rest days into your fitness routine are crucial strategies.

Supplements, while not a magic solution, can support your goals. For instance, whey protein can facilitate meeting your daily protein targets, and creatine has been shown to support strength and muscle mass retention during caloric restriction.

Remember, body recomposition—losing fat while preserving or gaining muscle—isn't a linear process. It requires patience, consistency, and the willingness to adjust your approach based on progress. Regular check-ins with yourself or a professional can help in fine-tuning your strategy for optimal results.

Ultimately, the journey towards fat loss and muscle preservation is highly personal. Factors such as genetics, starting point, and individual reactions to diet and exercise mean that what works for one person might not work for another. Hence, the importance of an experimental mindset, guided by best practices but adapted to your unique circumstances, cannot be overstressed.

By treating this process as a learning journey about your body, fostering self-discipline, and applying scientific principles, you can achieve sustainable fat loss while preserving, or even building, muscle mass. The key lies in understanding and applying the principles of a caloric deficit thoughtfully and strategically, ensuring that every calorie, every meal, and every workout moves you closer to your goal.

Meal Timing and Frequency for Optimising Fat Loss and Muscle Gain

Mastering the rhythm of when to eat and how often can significantly leverage your efforts in shedding fat and accruing muscle. The strategic deployment of meal timing and frequency emerges not just as a mere suggestion but as a critical component in sculpting an enviable physique. Let's simplify the complexity surrounding this topic, drawing upon the latest scientific insights, ensuring that every calorie and every protein gram you consume is put to optimal use.

The conventional wisdom of eating three square meals a day or the more modern approach of grazing on six smaller meals has been a topic of debate among fitness enthusiasts and researchers alike. However, evidence suggests that for those dedicated to fat loss while preserving lean muscle mass, the focal point shouldn't just be on *what* you eat but *when* and *how often*. This approach, when executed correctly, can positively influence your metabolic rate and hormone levels, which are catalysts in the body's fat-burning and muscle-building processes.

Intermittent fasting has surged in popularity, not just as a diet trend but as a scientifically backed method to enhance fat loss and muscle synthesis. By cycling periods of eating with periods of fasting, the body is forced to dip into its fat reserves for energy, thus driving fat loss. Concurrently, the growth hormone spikes observed in fasting states can aid in muscle preservation and growth, making it a potentially potent strategy for those looking to transform their body composition.

Yet, for building muscle, there's an important window that mustn't be ignored: the post-workout period. Consuming protein together with carbs within a 45-60-minute window after resistance training is important for kick-starting the muscle repair and growth process. This strategy, known as nutrient timing, leverages the body's heightened responsiveness to protein synthesis post-exercise, a factor that can significantly impact muscle gains over time.

When you are on a diet, it is important to consume a big portion of your calories around your training. Additionally, you should aim to consume 50% of your daily carbohydrate intake around the time of your training. This strategy helps in two ways. Firstly, it optimizes recovery after exercise, and secondly, it helps you consume fewer carbohydrates during the rest of the day while maintaining stable blood sugar levels, which is important for losing fat.

Post weight training, consuming an optimal ratio of carbohydrates and protein is crucial for recovery, muscle repair, and growth. The recommended amounts can vary based on the intensity and duration of the workout, as well as individual goals and dietary needs. However, general guidelines can help most individuals maximize their recovery and gains.

Protein Amount: It's recommended to consume about 20-40 grams of protein after training. This range is considered effective for stimulating muscle protein synthesis (MPS), the process that helps repair and build muscle tissue. **Why:** The amino acids in protein are the building blocks of muscle. Consuming protein post-workout supplies these essential nutrients, facilitating the repair of microtears in muscle fibers incurred during weight training. This not only aids in recovery but also contributes to muscle hypertrophy (growth).

Carbohydrates Amount: The recommended carbohydrate intake post-workout can vary widely, with a general guideline of 0.5-0.7 grams of carbohydrates per pound of body weight (1.1-1.5 grams/kg) within 30 minutes to an hour after exercise. **Why:** Carbohydrates are crucial for replenishing the muscle glycogen that has been depleted during your workout. Glycogen is the primary energy source for muscles during high-intensity activities, and replenishing it is essential for recovery and for ensuring that your muscles have the energy needed for subsequent workouts. Additionally, consuming carbohydrates in conjunction with protein can enhance the role of insulin in transporting amino acids into muscle cells, further promoting muscle repair and growth.

Combining Carbs and Protein Synergy: The combination of carbs and protein post-workout is more effective than consuming either macronutrient alone. This synergy enhances glycogen storage and protein synthesis more effectively than just protein or carbohydrates in isolation. **Practical Example:** A post-workout meal or shake that includes both carbohydrates and protein might look like a protein shake made with a banana and whey protein, or a whey protein shake with a quick acting carb like Highly Branched Cyclic Dextrin or dextrose.

However, it's not just about the post-workout meal. The frequency of protein intake throughout the day also plays a significant role in muscle synthesis. Distributing protein intake evenly across meals can maximize muscle protein synthesis rates, ensuring that the body has a continuous supply of amino acids to repair and build muscle tissue. For individuals focused on muscle gain, aiming for a protein-rich meal or snack every 3-4 hours is a wise tactic.

It's important, however, to tailor these strategies to individual lifestyles and preferences. The effectiveness of meal timing and frequency can vary based on personal schedules, daily energy expenditure, and even genetic predispositions. Experimentation and careful monitoring of progress are key in identifying what works best for your body.

Remember, the journey to an extraordinary physique is not solely defined by the hours spent lifting weights or pounding the pavement; it's equally about understanding the nuances of nutrition. Mastering meal timing and frequency can elevate your efforts, transforming your diet from a mere support act to a headline performer in achieving your fitness goals.

Supplements: What Works, What Doesn't, and What's Worth Considering

In the journey towards achieving an ideal body composition—stripping fat while preserving or even gaining muscle—the conversation inevitably swings towards supplements. With the supplement industry booming, it's crucial to separate the wheat from the chaff, discerning what genuinely aids your fitness goals from what's merely a hype-fueled money sink.

Protein powder: First off, let's talk protein supplements. They're the most talked-about, and for good reason. Protein is pivotal for muscle repair and growth. Studies consistently show that supplementing with protein, especially whey protein, can significantly enhance muscle protein synthesis, aiding in both recovery and muscle building. For those struggling to meet their protein requirements through diet alone, shakes can be a practical solution. A good tip to never miss a meal is having a couple of unmixed proteinshakes at work or in your or car all the time with a bottle of water. Unmixed you can keep them until needed.

Creatine: is another heavy-hitter in the supplement world, backed by a mountain of research attesting to its effectiveness in improving strength, power, and muscle mass. It's one of the few supplements that can claim to offer noticeable performance improvements, particularly in high-intensity activities and strength training.

How Creatine Works Energy Production: Creatine's primary role is to increase the availability of creatine phosphate in the muscles. Creatine phosphate helps regenerate ATP (adenosine triphosphate), which is the most basic form of energy used by cells. During high-intensity, short-duration exercises like weightlifting or sprinting, ATP is depleted quickly. By increasing creatine phosphate stores, creatine supplementation allows for more rapid ATP regeneration, which can lead to improved performance, enabling athletes to lift heavier weights, perform more repetitions, or sprint at a faster pace.

Cell Hydration: Creatine increases water content within muscle cells, a process known as cell volumization. This can slightly increase the size of the muscle and, more importantly, may signal cellular pathways that lead to muscle growth.

Reduced Fatigue: Some research suggests that creatine can help reduce fatigue and increase endurance, although its effects are most pronounced in short bursts of high-intensity activity.

Muscle Protein Synthesis: While creatine itself doesn't directly increase muscle protein synthesis, the increased workout capacity and cell signaling effects can contribute to muscle growth over time.

The most researched and recommended form of creatine is creatine monohydrate. It's effective, safe, and typically more affordable than other forms. Try to use 3-5 grams per day, preferably 30-60 min before a workout. And on non workout days take it with your morning meal as it also may have cognitive functions. Research suggests that creatine supplementation can have several cognitive benefits, especially in situations where the brain's energy demands are increased:

Improved Memory and Attention: Studies have shown that creatine can improve short-term memory and reduce mental fatigue. This is particularly evident in demanding cognitive tasks and under conditions of sleep deprivation or stress. **Enhanced Cognitive Performance:** Creatine supplementation may enhance overall cognitive performance, particularly in tasks that require speed of processing. Individuals following a vegetarian or vegan diet, who might have lower baseline creatine levels due to the absence of meat (a primary dietary source of creatine), can particularly benefit from supplementation.

Amino acids:

Branched-Chain Amino Acids (BCAAs) and Essential Amino Acids (EAAs) are crucial for muscle protein synthesis, recovery, and overall body composition, impacting both muscle gain and weight loss. Understanding their benefits and how to implement them can optimize your fitness results.

BCAAs: consist of three essential amino acids: leucine, isoleucine, and valine. They are termed "branched-chain" due to their chemical structure.

Benefits:

Muscle Protein Synthesis: Leucine, in particular, plays a significant role in initiating muscle protein synthesis, the process of building muscle tissue. **Reduced Exercise Fatigue:** BCAAs can help reduce the feeling of fatigue during exercise by influencing the production of serotonin in the brain. **Decreased Muscle Soreness:** They can reduce muscle damage and inflammation, leading to decreased soreness and faster recovery.

For Weight Loss: BCAAs may help preserve lean mass during a calorie deficit, ensuring that more of the weight lost comes from fat stores. This preservation of lean mass also helps maintain metabolic rate, crucial for long-term weight management.

For Muscle Gain: By stimulating muscle protein synthesis and aiding in recovery, BCAAs support the building of muscle. They're especially beneficial when consumed around the time of your workout.

EAAs: include the three BCAAs plus six other amino acids that the body cannot produce on its own and must be obtained through diet: histidine, lysine, methionine, phenylalanine, threonine, and tryptophan.

Benefits:

Complete Muscle Protein Synthesis: While BCAAs initiate the process, all nine EAAs are required to fully carry out muscle protein synthesis. **Enhanced Recovery and Performance:** EAAs support quicker recovery from exercise, reducing soreness and preparing the body for its next workout more effectively. **Supports Overall Health:** Beyond muscle, EAAs are essential for many bodily functions, including supporting the immune system, producing hormones, and aiding in various metabolic processes.

For Weight Loss: Similar to BCAAs, EAAs help preserve muscle mass during weight loss. The comprehensive support for muscle protein synthesis may be particularly beneficial when dietary protein intake is low.

For Muscle Gain: EAAs provide a more complete solution for muscle gain by supplying all the necessary building blocks for muscle protein synthesis. This can be especially important for maximizing gains from resistance training and other forms of exercise. How to Implement BCAAs and EAAs

Timing: Pre-Workout: Taking BCAAs or EAAs before workouts can provide energy to the muscles and may reduce fatigue, allowing for more intense training. **Post-Workout:** Consuming them after exercise can kickstart the recovery process, initiating muscle repair and growth. Dosage:

For BCAAs, a common dosage is 5-10 grams both before and after workouts. For EAAs, dosages vary but often range from 6-12 grams per serving, with similar timing to BCAAs.

Dietary Considerations: While supplements can be beneficial, especially around workouts or for those with higher requirements, getting a balanced intake of amino acids from high-quality protein sources throughout the day is also crucial for optimal health and performance. Integration into Diet:

Incorporate BCAAs or EAAs as part of a comprehensive nutrition plan that includes adequate protein, carbohydrates, and fats to support your fitness goals, whether for muscle gain, weight loss, or overall health. In summary, both BCAAs and EAAs offer benefits for muscle gain and weight loss by supporting muscle protein synthesis, reducing recovery time, and helping preserve lean muscle mass during calorie restriction. Proper timing and dosage can enhance their effectiveness, but they should complement a balanced diet and exercise program. Although i want to mention that if you already consume enough protein through foods this is not a game changer. But if youre on a strict diet they have their place.

Fat burners: Fat burners are where things get more contentious. The market is flooded with products claiming to boost metabolism, reduce appetite, or directly burn fat. Yet, the evidence supporting these claims is often thin. Caffeine is one of the few ingredients proven to enhance fat oxidation and can mildly increase metabolic rate, but its effects are modest at best. As for the rest, skepticism is warranted.

L-Carnitine: not a fat burner but more a fat transporter is an interesting naturally occurring amino acid derivative that's often taken as a weight loss supplement and is known for its role in energy production. It plays a crucial role in the metabolism of fat, serving as a transporter of fatty acids into the mitochondria, the engines within cells where these fats are burned for energy. This process not only helps the body produce energy but is also essential for muscle movement, heart and brain function, and numerous other body processes. Here's a closer look at its benefits, particularly regarding weight loss and muscle gain, and advice on supplementation.

Benefits of L-Carnitine Weight Loss: While L-Carnitine is marketed for its fat-burning capabilities, the evidence is mixed. Some studies suggest that it can aid weight loss by increasing the amount of fat burned during exercise and rest, potentially leading to improved fat loss over time. However, L-Carnitine is likely most effective when combined with a healthy diet and exercise program.

Exercise Performance: L-Carnitine supplementation has been linked to increased exercise performance. It can reduce fatigue and muscle soreness post-exercise, improve endurance by increasing oxygen supply to muscles, and reduce the production of lactic acid, which can hinder performance.

Muscle Gain: While L-Carnitine's direct role in muscle gain is less clear than its role in fat metabolism, it may contribute to muscle growth by reducing exercise-induced muscle damage, potentially leading to faster recovery times and improved performance over subsequent workouts.

How to Supplement with L-Carnitine Dosage: For weight loss and performance enhancement, doses of 500-2,000 mg per day are commonly recommended. It's worth noting that the effective dose can vary based on individual health status and goals.

Timing: Taking L-Carnitine with meals can enhance its absorption, as it may be better absorbed in the presence of dietary fats. However, specific timing for performance enhancement isn't as clearly defined and may depend on individual preferences or goals.

Form: L-Carnitine is available in several forms, including L-Carnitine L-Tartrate, Acetyl-L-Carnitine, and Propionyl-L-Carnitine. Acetyl-L-Carnitine is often used for cognitive benefits due to its ability to cross the blood-brain barrier, while L-Carnitine L-Tartrate is more commonly used for physical performance and recovery.

In summary, L-Carnitine can support weight loss and enhance exercise performance by improving fat metabolism and reducing exercise-induced muscle damage. However, its effectiveness can vary, and it should be used as a complement to, not a replacement for, a balanced diet and regular exercise.

The discussion wouldn't be complete without touching on the topic of multivitamins and omega-3 supplements. While not directly linked to fat loss or muscle gain, they play crucial roles in overall health and, by extension, your body's ability to perform and recover. For those whose diets lack nutritional variety, these supplements can help fill the gaps.

So, what's the takeaway? Focus on your diet first—the foundation of any successful fat loss and muscle preservation strategy. Supplements should complement, not replace, nourishing meals. If you choose to use supplements, prioritize those with solid scientific backing: protein, creatine, and perhaps caffeine and L-Carnitine for a pre-workout boost.

Remember, no supplement can outdo a poor diet or inconsistent training regime. Supplements might offer you a slight edge, but they're not shortcuts to an ideal body. It's your commitment to a well-rounded diet, consistent training, and a healthy lifestyle that will yield the most significant results.

Before adding any supplement to your regime, it's also crucial to consult with a healthcare provider, especially if you have underlying health conditions or are on medication. Safety first, always.

Lastly, embrace the process. Transforming your body is a journey requiring patience, hard work, and resilience. Supplements can be a valuable tool in your arsenal, but they're just one piece of the puzzle. Focus on nurturing your body with quality nutrition, pushing yourself in your workouts, and giving yourself ample time to rest and recover. That's the true blueprint for success.

Chapter 4:
Strength Training for
Optimal Body Recomposition

Achieving the perfect balance between shedding fat and preserving muscle requires a good understanding of nutrition and strength training. The principles of progressive overload, specificity, and recovery are the foundation of successful body recomposition. Strength training is an equally important part as nutrition that, when mastered, can improve your body's ability to burn fat and build muscle. By adopting the principles of strength training together with proper nutrition, you can reach your desired body recomposition goals with time.

Progressive overload, or gradually increasing the demands on your musculoskeletal system, is not just beneficial, it's essential for muscle growth. Specificity, the concept of tailoring your training towards very specific objectives, underscores the need for a well-structured strength training programme that aligns with your body recomposition goals. Similarly, recovery is not merely a break from training but a critical component of progress, allowing for muscle repair and growth.

Designing a strength training programme can seem daunting, but it begins with understanding and implementing a balance of compound and isolation exercises. Compound exercises, which engage multiple muscle groups, are your best ally in achieving more significant metabolic adaptions and muscle gains, while isolation exercises are valuable for targeting specific muscles that may need extra attention. A strategic blend of both, combined with the appropriate sets, reps, and rest, based on your individual progress, is important in crafting a body that's not just leaner, but stronger and more capable.

Strength training for optimal body recomposition is not about quick fixes but about steadfast dedication to intelligent, principled training. It's a powerful reminder that through consistent effort, the body's capacity for change is boundless. As you start on or continue your journey in strength training, remember that each session is a step toward not just a more aesthetically pleasing physique but a demonstration of personal strength, resilience, and the human potential for transformation. And dont forget a healthier and longer life.

Principles of Strength Training: Progressive Overload, Specificity, and Recovery

If you want to build muscle and lose fat through strength training, it's not just about lifting weights. You need to understand the principles of progressive overload, specificity, and recovery. These are essential for achieving the best results. Let's take a closer look at each of these principles and how you can incorporate them into your fitness routine.

To kick off, **progressive overload** is the bedrock of strength training. It's a simple yet profound concept suggesting that, to catalyse muscle growth, you must consistently increase the demands on your musculoskeletal system.

Progressive overload is a fundamental principle in strength training and physical fitness, emphasizing the importance of gradually increasing the demands on the musculoskeletal system to stimulate muscle growth, strength gains, and improvements in endurance. The concept is based on the idea that in order to improve, the body must be continually challenged with levels of stress or load that exceed what it has previously adapted to. This can be achieved through various methods, ensuring continuous progress and adaptation over time.

Ways to Implement Progressive Overload Increasing Weight: Perhaps the most straightforward method and always the one to start with, this involves adding more weight to an exercise over time. The goal is to gradually increase the weights lifted during each exercise by 2-5% every week. However, avoid increasing the weights before you reach your target maximum reps within your rep range for all of your sets for a specific exercise. For example, if you intend to do 3 sets of 12-15 reps of bench press, you should only increase the weight in the next session if you manage to achieve your target reps in all three sets during the current session, meaning you accomplished 15 reps for all three sets.

Increasing Repetitions: Another method is to increase the number of repetitions performed with a given weight. If you can perform 10 repetitions of a certain weight easily, try aiming for 11 or 12 repetitions with the same weight.

Increasing Volume: Volume is the total amount of work done, calculated as weight × sets × repetitions. Increasing any of these factors can increase the volume. For instance, adding an extra set to your workout increases the total volume.

Increasing Frequency: This involves increasing the number of training sessions for a particular muscle group within a given timeframe. For example, going from training legs once a week to twice a week.

Decreasing Rest Time: Shortening the rest intervals between sets can increase the intensity of the workout, forcing your body to work harder and adapt to a more demanding workload.

Improving Exercise Technique: Even without changing any other variable, simply improving the form or technique of an exercise can increase the effective load on the muscle, leading to better muscle activation and growth.

Changing Exercises: Incorporating new exercises or variations can challenge the muscles in different ways, contributing to continued growth and improvement.

Importance of Progressive Overload Muscle Growth and Strength: Progressive overload is crucial for hypertrophy (muscle growth) and strength gains because it challenges the muscles, leading to muscle fiber damage and subsequent repair and growth. **Avoiding Plateaus:** By continuously altering the training stimulus, you can avoid plateaus in performance and physique improvements. **Adaptation:** The body adapts to the stress placed upon it. Without progressively increasing the demand, improvements will stagnate as the body becomes efficient at handling the current stress level.

Considerations Recovery: Adequate rest and nutrition are essential for recovery and growth. Overloading without proper recovery can lead to overtraining, injury, and burnout. **Balance:** It's important to apply progressive overload in a balanced and structured manner to prevent imbalances or overuse injuries. **Individualization:** The application of progressive overload should be tailored to individual fitness levels, goals, and recovery capacities.

Moving on, **specificity** is about tailoring your workout regimen to align with your fitness goals. Essentially, it dictates that to excel in a particular area, your training must be directed and focused on that area. For example, if you're aiming for a marked improvement in squat strength, your program should prioritize movements that develop the muscle groups involved in squatting. This principle extends beyond just exercise selection; it encompasses workout structure, including volume and intensity pertinent to your objectives.

Furthermore, the role of **recovery** in strength training can't be overstated. It's the golden period when the magic of muscle repair and growth happens. Adequate rest, encompassing sleep and time between workout sessions, combined with proper nutrition, lays the foundation for effective recovery. Ignoring this principle can lead to overtraining, diminished performance, and even injuries, thereby jeopardizing your path to body recomposition.

Integrating these principles into your strength training regime necessitates a balanced approach. Progressive overload demands pushing your boundaries, yet it's crucial not to leap too far, too fast. Gradual increments in challenge ensure sustainable progress. And while pursuing those objectives with vigor, always carve out ample space for recovery, for it is in rest that you grow.

To craft a program that embodies these principles, start with a clear objective. Whether it's fat loss, muscle gain, or both, let that goal be the guiding light. From there, chart a course that progressively heightens the demands on your body, respects the specificity of your objectives, and incorporates strategic recovery periods. This could mean adjusting your workout volume, intensity, and frequency over time, always with an eye towards how your body responds.

It's also vital to listen to your body's feedback. Signs of excessive fatigue, lingering soreness, or halted progress are cues to reassess your training load, recovery adequacy, and whether your program is truly aligned with your goals. Adaptability, in response to your body's cues, is key to circumventing plateaus and ensuring continuous progress toward your body recomposition ambitions.

In practice, a well-rounded strength training plan might include a mix of compound and isolation exercises, varied rep ranges, and sufficient rest days. The inclusion of progressive overload can be achieved by increasing the weights lifted, enhancing the volume of workouts, or reducing rest intervals over time. Specificity is reflected in the choice of exercises and programming structure that align to the individual's goals, while recovery is facilitated through rest days, sleep quality, and nutrition.

The principles of progressive overload, specificity, and recovery are crucial for strength training. By mastering these principles, you can push your physical abilities to their limits and achieve your desired physique. This requires discipline, dedication, and a deep understanding of these tenets. Remember, success in strength training is inevitable if you follow these principles strictly.

Designing a Strength Training Programme: Exercises, Sets, Reps, and Rest

When it comes to reshaping your body through strength training, it's not just about lifting weights. It takes careful planning and understanding to succeed. The key to your success is a well-designed strength training program that aligns with your goals and keeps you progressing. This chapter will guide you in constructing a program that will help you achieve your goals efficiently and effectively.

First and foremost, selecting the right mix of exercises is important. Your programme should ideally encompass a balance of compound exercises—such as squats, deadlifts, and bench presses—which target multiple muscle groups, and isolation exercises, like bicep curls and triceps extensions, for targeting specific muscles. Compound exercises are particularly effective for stimulating muscle growth and boosting metabolic rate, thus playing a crucial role in body recomposition.

The number of sets and repetitions (reps) is another critical aspect that significantly influences your training outcomes. For beginners, starting with 8-12 sets per week per musclegroup of total volume and 8-12 reps per exercise is a recommended guideline that balances muscle growth and endurance build-up. As you progress, adjusting the sets and reps can help you break through plateaus and continue making gains. It's about finding what challenges you; if it doesn't challenge you, it won't change you.

Heres a few examples of how you could get started.

Beginner Program Total Sets Per Week Per Muscle Group: 8-12 **Reps Per Set:** 12-15 **Frequency:** 2-3 days per week for each muscle group **Intensity:** Light to moderate weights, focusing on mastering technique and form **Example Split:** Full body routines or upper/lower splits, ensuring all major muscle groups are worked within the week.

Example for Chest: Monday: Bench Press 3 sets of 12-15 reps, Dumbbell Flyes 3 sets of 12-15 reps Thursday: Push-ups 3 sets of 12-15 reps, Incline Dumbbell Press 3 sets of 12-15 reps

Intermediate Program Total Sets Per Week Per Muscle Group: 12-16 **Reps Per Set:** 8-12 **Frequency:** Increasing frequency to 3-4 days per week for each muscle group **Intensity:** Moderate weights, focusing on gradually increasing the weight while maintaining form **Example Split:** Push/Pull/Legs split or a more specialized split to allow increased focus on individual muscle groups.

Example for Chest: Monday (Push Day): Bench Press 4 sets of 8-12 reps, Incline Dumbbell Press 3 sets of 8-12 reps Thursday (Push Day): Dumbbell Flyes 4 sets of 8-12 reps, Cable Crossover 3 sets of 8-12 reps

Advanced Program Total Sets Per Week Per Muscle Group: 16-20+ **Reps Per Set:** Varies – 6-12 for hypertrophy, 1-5 for strength focus **Frequency:** 4-6 days per week, depending on split and recovery **Intensity:** High, with a focus on maximizing the load while employing advanced techniques (drop sets, supersets, etc.) **Example Split:** Specialized splits, allowing for targeted focus and increased volume per muscle group, or a more frequent push/pull/legs split done twice a week.

Example for Chest: Monday (Chest Day): Bench Press 4 sets of 6-8 reps, Incline Barbell Press 4 sets of 6-8 reps, Dumbbell Flyes 4 sets of 8-12 reps, Cable Crossover 3 sets of 12 reps (Drop Set on final set) Thursday (Upper Body Push Focus): Incline Dumbbell Press 4 sets of 8-10 reps, Machine Chest Press 3 sets of 10-12 reps, Push-ups 4 sets to failure

Progression Tips: Beginners should focus on learning proper form, gradually increasing weight as 15 reps become manageable. Intermediates can start manipulating variables more aggressively, adding weight, and experimenting with different rep ranges and volume. Advanced lifters should employ a variety of training techniques, including periodization, to continue making gains in strength and size, avoiding plateaus. Remember, these are starting points. Effective program design considers individual recovery ability, goals, and lifestyle factors. It's also crucial to include adequate rest, nutrition, and possibly periodization strategies to manage intensity and volume over time for sustained progress.

The structure of a weight training program can significantly affect its outcomes, targeting different goals such as muscle gain, fat loss, strength improvement, or overall fitness. Among the various training splits, three popular formats are the full-body workout, upper/lower split, and push/pull (often extended to push/pull/legs) split. Each has its advantages and suits different training levels, schedules, and goals.

Full-Body Workout Description: Full-body workouts involve exercises that target all major muscle groups within a single session. These workouts are typically performed several times a week with at least one day of rest in between.

Benefits: Comprehensive stimulation of all muscle groups within a single session. Higher frequency per muscle group without requiring daily gym visits. Efficient for those with limited time to dedicate to gym sessions.

Ideal For: Beginners to intermediate trainees who benefit from the high frequency of muscle stimulation. Individuals looking for a balanced approach to strength and muscle gain. Those with limited weekly availability to work out.

Upper/Lower Split Description: This split divides training sessions into upper body days and lower body days. Typically, this involves 4 days of training per week, allowing each muscle group to be worked twice.

Benefits: Allows for focused intensity on either the upper or lower body, leading to better recovery. Enables a higher weekly training volume since each muscle group is targeted more directly. Offers flexibility in arranging workouts and managing recovery. **Ideal For:** Intermediate to advanced trainees who require more volume and intensity to see progress. Those looking to increase muscle mass or strength with a moderate to high frequency. Individuals who can commit to 4 days of training per week.

Push/Pull/Legs Split Description: This split organizes workouts based on movement patterns: "push" exercises (e.g., bench press, shoulder press) that primarily utilize the chest, shoulders, and triceps; "pull" exercises (e.g., rows, pull-ups) for the back and biceps; and "legs" for lower body. This split can be run 3, 4, or 6 days a week, depending on whether legs are trained once or twice and if push/pull sessions are combined or separate.

Benefits: Highly specialized focus on specific muscle groups or movements. Allows for high volume and intensity, suitable for muscle hypertrophy and strength. Versatile in frequency adjustment, accommodating various commitment levels. **Ideal For:** Intermediate to advanced athletes focusing on muscle hypertrophy and strength. Those with the ability to train 3-6 days per week and looking to maximize muscle group focus. Individuals seeking to overcome plateaus by intensifying focus on specific muscle groups.

Choosing the right split depends on several factors including your training experience, goals, recovery capacity, and schedule. Full-body workouts are great for beginners and those with limited time, providing a foundation and stimulating overall muscle growth. Upper/lower splits offer a balanced approach for those ready to increase their training volume and intensity, while push/pull/legs splits cater to more experienced lifters aiming for maximal muscle hypertrophy and strength with focused and frequent training sessions. Ultimately, the best choice is the one that fits your lifestyle, allows for consistent progress, and keeps you motivated.

Among the most common misconceptions is the belief that more is always better. However, the science of muscle hypertrophy suggests a threshold beyond which additional volume does not equate to faster growth and might instead lead to overtraining. Listening to your body and allowing sufficient recovery time is paramount. Remember, muscles grow outside the gym when you're resting and refuelling.

Rest is a critical component of any effective workout routine, both in terms of rest between sets during a workout and rest days between workout sessions. Understanding the importance of rest can help optimize training results by balancing exercise with recovery to promote muscle growth, strength gains, and overall fitness improvement.

Rest Between Sets Energy Recovery: Adequate rest between sets allows for partial replenishment of ATP (adenosine triphosphate) and creatine phosphate, the primary energy sources used during high-intensity, short-duration exercises. This replenishment helps maintain the quality and intensity of your performance throughout the workout.

Lactic Acid Clearance: Resting between sets helps in the removal of lactic acid produced during anaerobic exercise, reducing muscle fatigue and soreness, which can improve endurance and performance in subsequent sets.

Muscle Recovery: Short recovery periods between sets can also prevent excessive muscle fatigue, allowing for better maintenance of technique and reducing the risk of injury.

Training Goals Adaptation: The optimal rest period between sets can vary based on your training objectives. For strength and power, longer rest periods (2-5 minutes) are typically recommended to allow for maximal effort in each set. For hypertrophy (muscle growth), slightly shorter rest periods (1-2 minutes) are often used to create a balance between intensity and volume with a moderate level of fatigue. For endurance training, even shorter rest periods (<1 minute) are utilized to enhance cardiovascular and muscular endurance.

Rest Days Between Workouts Muscle Repair and Growth: Exercise, especially resistance training, creates micro-tears in muscle fibers. Rest days are crucial for allowing these fibers to repair and grow stronger. Muscle growth occurs outside the gym during recovery periods, not during the exercise itself.

Prevention of Overtraining: Regular rest days prevent overtraining syndrome, characterized by a plateau or decline in performance, increased risk of injury, and psychological stress. Adequate rest ensures the nervous system, muscles, and connective tissues have sufficient time to recover.

Replenishment of Energy Stores: Rest days allow for the replenishment of glycogen stores in the muscles and liver, which are depleted during exercise. This replenishment is vital for maintaining energy levels and performance in subsequent workouts.

Psychological Recovery: Rest days help prevent burnout and maintain motivation by providing a mental break from the rigors of continuous training, which is essential for long-term adherence to any fitness program.

Incorporating appropriate rest intervals between sets and ensuring adequate rest days between workouts are fundamental for achieving optimal performance, progression, and overall health. Balancing exercise with sufficient recovery enables the body to repair, adapt, and grow stronger, highlighting the importance of rest as an integral part of any successful training routine. Tailoring rest periods to individual needs, training intensity, and specific goals can further enhance the benefits of rest in promoting progression and achieving fitness objectives.

Lastly, credibility and information quality cannot be overstated. Relying on evidence-based practices and continuously educating yourself or seeking guidance from certified professionals ensures that your strength training programme isn't just a routine but a sustainable, evolving path to peak physical form and beyond.

Compound vs. Isolation Exercises for Maximum Efficiency

When planning a workout routine for maximum efficiency, understanding the distinction between compound and isolation exercises is crucial. Both types of exercises serve important roles in a fitness program, but they have different impacts on the body and are used for different purposes.

Compound Exercises Definition: Compound exercises involve multiple joints and muscle groups working together during the movement. These exercises are efficient for building strength and muscle mass, improving athletic performance, and burning more calories due to the larger amount of muscle involved.

Examples: Squats, deadlifts, bench presses, and pull-ups.

Benefits:

Efficiency: Because they work multiple muscle groups at once, you can get a full-body workout with fewer exercises, making your training sessions more time-effective. **Functional Strength:** They mimic real-world movements and activities, helping improve functional strength and performance in daily tasks or sports. **Increased Caloric Burn:** Engaging multiple muscle groups simultaneously requires more energy, thus burning more calories during and after the workout. **Greater Hormonal Response:** Compound exercises are known to induce a more significant release of muscle-building hormones like testosterone and growth hormone.

Isolation Exercises Definition: Isolation exercises target a single joint and muscle group at a time. These are particularly useful for focusing on specific muscles to shape or strengthen them, rehabilitating injured areas, or correcting muscle imbalances.

Examples: Bicep curls, tricep extensions, leg curls, and calf raises.

Benefits:

Targeted Muscle Development: Allows for focused work on a particular muscle to increase its size and strength, which is beneficial for bodybuilding or addressing weaknesses. **Rehabilitation:** Ideal for rehabilitating after injuries, as they can isolate and strengthen injured or weakened areas without placing undue stress on other body parts. **Muscle Imbalances:** Useful for correcting imbalances by strengthening smaller or weaker muscles that may not be adequately engaged during compound movements.

For Maximum Efficiency Foundation with Compound Exercises: For most individuals, especially those with limited time, focusing on compound exercises can provide comprehensive benefits in terms of strength, muscle mass, and caloric expenditure. They should form the core of your workout program.

Detailing with Isolation Exercises: Isolation exercises can then be used to target specific muscles that need extra attention, whether for aesthetic purposes, strength imbalances, or rehabilitation.

Balanced Approach: Incorporating both types of exercises in a balanced manner can maximize efficiency by ensuring the development of overall strength and muscle mass while also allowing for focused improvements on specific muscle groups.

Personalization: Tailor your blend of compound and isolation exercises to fit your fitness goals, whether it's bodybuilding, strength, general fitness, or rehabilitation. For example, bodybuilders may place more emphasis on isolation exercises to sculpt particular muscles, while athletes might prioritize compound movements to improve overall performance.

For maximum efficiency in a workout program, leverage the broad, functional benefits of compound exercises as the foundation of your routine, supplemented by isolation exercises to target specific muscles for balanced development and aesthetic refinement. This approach ensures comprehensive strength and muscle gains while also addressing individual goals and needs.

The synergy between compound and isolation exercises cannot be overstated. Integrating both types into a strength training routine ensures comprehensive muscular development and efficient fat loss. Compound exercises build a solid foundation of strength and mass, while isolation exercises contribute to the refinement and balance of the physique. This holistic approach accelerates the body recomposition process, making the journey towards reaching fitness goals more streamlined and effective.

From a scientific standpoint, the combination of these exercises supports the principle of 'muscular confusion,' which posits that constantly varying exercises and the muscles being targeted can prevent plateaus in strength gains and fat loss. It's not about tricking the muscles, as some suggest, but rather about ensuring all muscle fibers are engaged over time, supporting consistent progress.

Moreover, the compatibility between compound and isolation exercises is evident in their contribution to enhancing one's functional strength and day-to-day performance. Compound movements improve overall body mechanics and coordination, which, when complemented with the precision of isolation exercises, result in a well-rounded athleticism. This dual approach not only aids in achieving an aesthetically pleasing physique but also enhances the quality of life by improving physical abilities.

However, it is essential to tailor the balance of compound and isolation exercises to one's individual goals, current fitness level, and any existing imbalances or injuries. Maintaining a focus on proper form and technique, especially in compound movements, is crucial to prevent injuries and ensure the effectiveness of the exercises. The complexity of these movements necessitates a keen attention to detail, as improper execution can lead to strain and counterproductive outcomes. Seeking guidance from a certified fitness professional can be invaluable in mastering these exercises.

How to Adapt Your Training Programme as You Progress

It's crucial to understand that the path ahead is not a linear one. Your body is a dynamic organism, constantly adapting to the demands placed upon it. This means that the training programme which initially challenges you will, over time, become less effective as your body becomes more efficient. The key to sustained progress, then, is in adapting your training regime as you advance.

Adaptation in strength training is guided by the principle of progressive overload, the idea being to gradually increase the weight, frequency, or intensity of your workouts to challenge your muscles in new ways. This might mean changing up your sets and reps, trying different exercises, or incorporating advanced training techniques like supersets or drop sets. This ongoing process of fine-tuning is essential for breaking through plateaus and achieving continuous improvement.

However, adaptation isn't just about pushing harder; it's equally important to ensure your body gets adequate rest and recovery between workouts. As you progress, your training sessions will likely become more intense, demanding more from your body. It's during rest that your muscles repair and grow stronger, so ignoring recovery can lead to overtraining and stall your progress.

Understanding the science of muscle hypertrophy can also guide your programme adaptations. Studies demonstrate that both mechanical tension and muscle damage contribute to muscle growth. As such, incorporating a variety of exercises that place the muscles under tension in different ways can enhance your gains. This could mean varying your grip or stance on certain exercises from one training block to the next, or incorporating a mixture of both compound and isolation movements throughout your programme.

Frequent assessment and adaptation of your training programme are essential. Every 2-3 weeks, evaluate your progress against your goals. Are you getting stronger? Are your muscles growing? If your progress is stalling, it might be time to adjust your routine. Regular adjustments keep your body guessing and progressing. Additionally, as your body changes, so too might your goals. What started as a mission for fat loss might evolve into a desire for muscle definition or increased strength, necessitating programme adjustments. Although all adjustments should start with progressing your lifts through progressive overload. Changing your entire program might be something you look at every 6 months or even less.

Listening to your body is paramount. While it's important to push yourself, recognising the signs of overtraining and giving your body the rest it needs is equally important. If you're constantly sore, feeling fatigued, or your performance is declining, these could be signs that your body needs a break. Scaling back or taking a few days off can sometimes be the best way to move forward.

Nutrition also plays a crucial role in how you adapt your training programme. As you progress and your body composition changes, your nutritional needs will evolve. Increased muscle mass means your body will burn more calories at rest, potentially increasing your calorie needs. Conversely, if fat loss is your goal, creating and adjusting to the right caloric deficit while ensuring adequate protein intake is key to preserving muscle mass.

Another aspect of adaptation is the incorporation of new methodologies and technologies into your training. Whether it's using apps to track your workouts and progress or incorporating wearable technology to monitor your physiological responses during exercise, these tools can provide invaluable feedback, helping you to make more informed decisions about when and how to adapt your training programme.

To sum it up, the journey to optimal body recomposition is a dynamic one, requiring a flexible and adaptive approach to strength training. By understanding the principles of progressive overload, the importance of recovery, and the role of nutrition, and by being attuned to your body's feedback, you can continuously evolve your training programme to meet your changing needs and goals. Remember, progress in strength training is a testament to your commitment to constantly challenge yourself while listening and adapting to your body's needs.

Adapt, evolve, and overcome – the path to your best self is through persistent effort and mindful adjustments to your training programme.

Chapter 5:
Cardiovascular Exercise in Body Recomposition

Cardiovascular exercise is an essential component of any fitness routine, especially for those looking to achieve a sculpted physique. When combined with strength training, cardio can help with both fat loss and muscle preservation. But what exactly does cardio do for the body, and how can one best incorporate it into their workout regimen?

First and foremost, cardio helps to improve heart health and boost metabolic efficiency. Additionally, when executed with precision, it can safeguard against muscle catabolism, which is often a concern when in a calorie-deficient state. The key to unlocking the full potential benefits of cardio lies in the balance between the intensity and duration of cardiovascular activities.

High-Intensity Interval Training (HIIT) has been praised in the scientific community for its superior efficacy in burning fat while maintaining a metabolic milieu favorable for muscle preservation. This form of cardio involves bursts of maximal effort followed by brief recovery periods, making it an excellent option for those who are short on time but still want to see results.

On the flip side, steady-state cardio, which is often perceived as the traditional route to fat loss, retains its relevance, particularly for those seeking a less demanding, yet effective, method for calorie expenditure. But it's not just about the type of cardio you choose - it's also important to balance cardio with strength training to prevent overtraining and ensure that muscle synthesis rates remain unimpeded.

Incorporating cardio into your fitness routine can help improve heart health, boost metabolic efficiency, and safeguard against muscle catabolism. High-Intensity Interval Training (HIIT) and steady-state cardio are both effective options, and balancing cardio with strength training is key to achieving optimal results.

The Role of Cardio in Fat Loss

On our way towards achieving the perfect blend of muscle gain and fat loss, cardiovascular exercise, or cardio, is important. While strength training builds the foundation for muscle mass and boosts metabolism, cardio accelerates the fat loss process, creating the deficit needed for your body to tap into fat stores for energy. Understanding the mechanics of how cardio aids in fat loss, alongside its integration into a comprehensive body recomposition strategy, can significantly enhance your results.

At its core, fat loss boils down to energy balance – consuming fewer calories than you burn. While diet plays the dominant role in establishing a caloric deficit, cardio has the dual benefit of increasing the caloric expenditure while potentially improving your cardiovascular health. Whether it's a fiery session of high-intensity interval training (HIIT) or a prolonged steady-state jog, your choice of cardio should align with your fitness level, preferences, and overall body recomposition goals.

The beauty of cardio in the context of fat loss is its versatility. HIIT, for instance, has been shown to offer superior benefits in a shorter timeframe, boosting both calorie burn and metabolic rate post-exercise. This is not to discredit the value of steady-state cardio, which is more accessible for beginners and those with joint issues, also contributing significantly to total calorie burn and endurance enhancement.

Moreover, cardio isn't just a tool for creating a caloric deficit but is instrumental in preserving lean muscle mass during a cut. When complemented with strength training and adequate protein intake, aerobic exercises contribute to a more favourable body fat to muscle ratio, ensuring that what you lose is predominantly fat, not muscle.

However, the implementation of cardio in a fat loss regimen must be strategic. An excessive volume or intensity of cardio can lead to overtraining, increased appetite, and potential loss of muscle if not balanced with strength training and proper nutrition. It's about finding that sweet spot where cardio serves its purpose without undermining muscle preservation and overall recovery.

Another often overlooked aspect of cardio is its ability to enhance your psychological well-being. Regular aerobic exercise has been associated with reductions in stress, anxiety, and depression, all of which can be barriers to consistent training and diet adherence. Thus, incorporating cardio into your routine not only aids in physical transformation but fortifies your mental resilience, keeping you focused and motivated on your body recomposition journey.

Practically, integrating cardio doesn't have to be daunting. Starting with as little as 20 to 30 minutes of low to moderate-intensity cardio 3 to 4 times a week can yield significant benefits. The key is consistency and progression; as your fitness improves, you can increase either the duration or intensity of your cardio sessions, tailored to your evolving fitness goals and preferences.

Ultimately, cardio should not be viewed in isolation but as a critical component of a comprehensive body recomposition strategy that includes strength training, nutrition, and recovery. It's the synergy among these elements that catalyses fat loss, muscle preservation, and overall health improvement.

The role of cardio in fat loss is undeniably significant. Its direct impact on energy expenditure, alongside benefits like muscle preservation, cardiovascular health, and mental well-being, makes it an indispensable tool in your fitness arsenal. Embrace cardio not as a monotonous obligation but as an activity that takes you closer to your body recomposition goals.

High-Intensity Interval Training (HIIT) vs. Steady-State Cardio: Benefits and When to Use Each

Understanding the roles of different forms of cardiovascular exercise cannot be overstated. High-Intensity Interval Training (HIIT) and steady-state cardio stand out as two important pillars for fat loss and muscle maintenance. Both hold unique benefits, and strategic implementation of each can catalyse your transformation.

HIIT, characterised by short bursts of intense activity followed by rest or low-intensity periods, has been lauded for its efficiency. A study by Gibala et al. (2012) illustrates that HIIT can enhance aerobic capacity comparably to traditional endurance training in a fraction of the time. This makes HIIT an appealing option for those with time constraints, seeking to maximise fat loss while preserving lean muscle mass. The high intensity of the workouts increases the metabolic rate post-exercise more significantly than steady-state cardio, a phenomenon known as 'afterburn' or excess post-exercise oxygen consumption (EPOC).

Steady-state cardio, on the other hand, is defined by maintaining a consistent pace at a moderate intensity for an extended period. It's the marathon runner's approach to cardiovascular health, building endurance and aiding in the recovery process by enhancing blood flow and reducing muscle soreness. Its benefits extend to improving cardiovascular health, with a lower risk of injury compared to high-impact HIIT workouts. For individuals new to exercise or those with specific health considerations, steady-state cardio can be a safer, more manageable starting point.

So, when should you use HIIT vs. steady-state cardio? The answer lies in your personal fitness goals and current physical condition. HIIT is particularly effective for fat loss, improving aerobic and anaerobic fitness, and saving time. It's suited for those who are already somewhat active and looking to push their limits. However, due to its intensity, it's crucial to incorporate adequate rest and recovery to prevent overtraining and injury.

Steady-state cardio, while potentially less efficient for fat loss, is invaluable for building a solid aerobic base, which in turn can support recovery from more strenuous workouts. It's ideal for endurance athletes or those who enjoy longer sessions of physical activity. Additionally, for individuals targeting specific heart rate zones to enhance fat burning or cardiovascular health, steady-state cardio offers controlled and sustained effort. Steady-state cardio can be more muscle sparing than HIIT, making it particularly important to preserve glycogen stores for your gym sessions.

Incorporating a mix of HIIT and steady-state cardio into your fitness routine can help you achieve maximum fat loss and improve cardiovascular health and endurance. You can mitigate the risks of overtraining by combining HIIT and steady-state workouts throughout the week, while still reaping the benefits of both workout styles.

Beyond the physical benefits, the psychological impacts of varying your workout routine cannot be overlooked. Incorporating both HIIT and steady-state cardio keeps workouts interesting and challenging, reducing the likelihood of boredom and enhancing adherence to a long-term fitness regime.

To sum it up, both HIIT and steady-state cardio have distinctive roles in body recomposition, with each offering unique advantages. Their optimal use hinges on individual goals, preferences, and physical condition.

Balancing Cardio with Strength Training to Avoid Muscle Loss

Blending cardio with strength training is not merely a strategy but a necessity. While cardio workouts undoubtedly play a role in fat loss, striking the right balance with strength training ensures that muscle mass isn't compromised in the process. This concept is fundamental for anyone keen on sculpting a physique that's not just lean, but also muscular and strong.

Cardiovascular exercise, known for its fat-burning efficiency, can, when overdone or improperly balanced with resistance training, lead to a decrease in muscle mass. This is a scenario you want to avoid at all costs. The key lies in integrating cardio in such a way that complements, rather than detracts from, your strength training efforts. This approach cultivates an environment within your body that favours fat loss while preserving hard-earned muscle.

Strength training, on the other hand, is the cornerstone of muscle preservation and growth. Through resistance training, you not only increase your muscle size but also enhance your metabolic rate, which in turn aids in burning more fat, even when you're not actively working out. It's a virtuous cycle that feeds into your body recomposition goals. The principle of progressive overload ensures that your muscles continue to adapt and grow stronger over time, offsetting any potential muscle loss from cardio exercises.

To achieve the ideal balance, it's crucial to tailor your cardio sessions to support your strength goals. High-Intensity Interval Training (HIIT) is particularly effective when paired with a strength training regimen. HIIT sessions, known for their short bursts of intense activity followed by rest or low-intensity intervals, can enhance endurance and fat oxidation without the prolonged catabolic states often induced by extended periods of steady-state cardio. This form of cardio has been shown to be particularly synergistic with strength training, facilitating improved muscle retention and fat loss.

Frequency, intensity, and timing are critical factors in balancing your cardio with strength training. A practical approach is to alternate your days between cardio and strength training, allowing for ample recovery and growth periods. For those who prefer coupling both on the same day, it's generally advised to prioritise strength training before cardio to optimise energy levels and performance for lifting. This strategy ensures that your muscle endurance and strength are not compromised by prior exhaustive cardio.

Exercising in the correct order can significantly impact your workout results, particularly when balancing cardio and strength training. The reason you might not want to perform cardio before strength training is largely due to how it affects muscle-building processes, particularly the activation of the mammalian target of rapamycin (mTOR) pathway.

The mTOR pathway is a crucial cellular mechanism that regulates muscle growth. It responds to various stimuli, including mechanical stress (like lifting weights) and nutritional status. When activated, mTOR signals the body to synthesize protein, leading to muscle repair and growth. This pathway is especially responsive following resistance or strength training exercises.

Here's why performing cardio before strength training can be counterproductive in terms of maximizing muscle growth and mTOR activation:

Energy Depletion: Cardiovascular exercise consumes glycogen stored in your muscles for energy. If you deplete a significant portion of this energy before lifting weights, your muscles might not have enough fuel to perform at peak levels during strength training. This reduced intensity may lead to a less effective stimulus for mTOR activation and muscle growth.

Fatigue and Performance: Cardio before strength training can lead to muscle fatigue. When muscles are already tired from cardio, your ability to lift heavy weights and maintain the intensity needed for optimal muscle growth is compromised. Lower intensity and volume in strength training mean less activation of the mTOR pathway.

Hormonal Impact: Exercise influences hormone levels, including cortisol and testosterone. Intense or prolonged cardio can increase cortisol levels, which might have a catabolic effect, potentially hindering muscle growth by affecting the mTOR pathway negatively. On the other hand, strength training increases testosterone levels, which can synergize with mTOR to promote muscle growth if strength training is not preceded by exhaustive cardio.

Interference Effect: There is a concept known as the "interference effect," where doing endurance and strength training in close succession may impair the muscle-building response. While the exact mechanisms are complex, part of this effect could be due to the conflicting signals sent to muscle cells from both types of exercises. Endurance training might activate pathways that work in opposition to the mTOR pathway, thus reducing its effectiveness for muscle growth.

For optimal results, it's generally recommended to separate cardio and strength training sessions if possible or to perform strength training before cardio within the same session. This approach prioritizes mTOR activation and muscle growth from strength training while still incorporating the cardiovascular benefits of aerobic exercise. However, individual goals, preferences, and recovery capabilities should always guide exercise sequencing decisions.

Nutrition also plays a an important role. Ensuring adequate protein intake supports muscle repair and growth, essential for offsetting any muscle protein breakdown that may occur during cardio activities. Carbohydrates are equally important, as they replenish muscle glycogen stores depleted during both strength and cardio sessions, fuelling your workouts and recovery. Having som sugars in the form of cyclic dextrin or dextrose in you water may help if you need to do both cardio and strenght session at the same time.

Monitoring your overall progress is key. If you notice a decline in strength or muscle size, it might be a sign that your cardio is overshadowing your strength training, calling for an adjustment in your regimen. Listening to your body and being responsive to its feedback is fundamental in fine-tuning the balance between cardio and strength training.

To achieve a balanced body composition, it's important to balance cardio and strength training. This can be achieved through a well-planned approach that includes HIIT, proper scheduling, good nutrition, and regular progress tracking. With these elements in place, it's possible to lose fat while maintaining and even building muscle mass. This approach is key to achieving and maintaining a healthy and optimal body composition.

Chapter 6:
Rest, Recovery, and Muscle Growth

When it comes to building a transformed, muscular physique, the grind of the workout itself is only half the battle. The other half lies in giving your body enough time to rest and recover. Rest and recovery are the foundation upon which muscle growth is built. Without sufficient time and conditions for muscle repair, your progress will stall.

It's important to understand that every training session causes your muscles to tear, which then triggers your body's natural repair process. But this repair process only leads to muscle hypertrophy when given the proper time and conditions. These conditions include adequate sleep and stress management, which are both essential for muscle growth.

Neglecting rest and recovery can be detrimental to your progress. If you don't allow your muscles enough time to repair, you risk not only stalling your progress but also increasing your risk of injury. Over time, this can lead to burnout and frustration.

Remember that rest and recovery are just as important as the workout itself. Don't underestimate the power of adequate sleep and recovery strategies, as they are key to reaching your fitness goals and achieving the transformed physique you desire.

Effective stress management is crucial for muscle recovery and growth. High cortisol levels can hinder recovery, but practices such as mindfulness, yoga, or breathing exercises can help reduce stress levels. Recovery isn't just about bouncing back; it's about creating a thriving environment for growth. Remember, what you do outside the gym is just as important as what you do inside it when it comes to transformation.

The Importance of Rest and Sleep in Muscle Recovery and Growth

When it comes to achieving fitness goals, rest and sleep are often overlooked but they are actually critical to muscle recovery and growth. In fact, they are just as important as your workouts and diet plans. Without adequate rest, your body won't be able to fully recover from the stress of exercise and you may even experience a decline in performance. So make sure to prioritize rest and sleep as part of your fitness routine for optimal results.

Sleep isn't just downtime. It's the golden period when the magic of muscle repair, growth, and strengthening occurs. During sleep, the body enters into a state of anabolic growth, where it repairs the micro-damage inflicted on muscle fibres during strength training. This process is crucial for muscle hypertrophy and in ensuring that muscles come back stronger post-workout.

Moreover, sleep profoundly affects hormonal balance, which in turn impacts muscle recovery and growth. During deep sleep, the human growth hormone (HGH) is released in pulses. This hormone plays a pivotal role in muscle growth and fat loss. Inadequate sleep can disrupt this hormonal balance, leading to decreased HGH levels, which can hamper muscle recovery and growth, and potentially lead to an increase in fat storage.

Another aspect often overlooked is the impact of sleep on performance. A well-rested body and mind can perform at peak levels, allowing for more intense and productive workouts. Conversely, sleep deprivation can lead to a decrease in physical performance, including reduced strength, slower reaction times, and diminished endurance, all of which can limit the effectiveness of your training sessions.

Rest days are equally important for muscle recovery and growth. Rest days allow muscles to repair, rebuild, and strengthen. Additionally, these days serve to replenish glycogen stores, reduce the risk of overtraining, and prevent mental burnout. Implementing rest days in your fitness regime ensures that both your body and mind have the necessary time to recover and prepare for the challenges ahead.

It's during rest periods that the body adapts to the stress of exercise. This adaptation process enhances muscular endurance and strength over time. Neglecting rest can lead to overtraining syndrome, characterized by a plateau in performance and possibly regression in strength and endurance. Overtraining not only stalls progress but also increases the risk of injury, which could set you back significantly.

But how much sleep do we really need for optimal recovery and muscle growth? While individual needs may vary, the general consensus points towards 7-9 hours of quality sleep per night for most adults. Quality here implies uninterrupted sleep, which allows the body to cycle through all stages of sleep, including the rapid eye movement (REM) phase, which is crucial for cognitive functions and overall recovery.

Creating a conducive sleep environment can significantly enhance sleep quality. This can be achieved by maintaining a cool, dark, and quiet bedroom. Reducing exposure to screens and blue light before bedtime can also help in improving sleep quality, as blue light has been shown to disrupt natural sleep patterns.

So, in the quest for muscle growth and fat loss, make rest and sleep your allies. By prioritising these often-neglected aspects of recovery, you're not just giving your body the chance to grow and strengthen, but also equipping it to tackle more rigorous workouts and overcome plateaus, propelling you towards your fitness goals with greater vigour and resilience.

In essence, treat rest and sleep with the same reverence you do your workouts and nutrition. This holistic approach is a surefire way to not only achieve but also sustain your body composition goals, turning fitness into a sustainable lifestyle rather than a transient phase. So, as you push your limits, remember, growth happens not just in the gym, but in the quiet moments of rest that follow.

Strategies for Effective Recovery

Recovery stands as the cornerstone that many overlook. It's in the rest periods, when muscles rebuild stronger and more resilient, that true transformation occurs. The strategies for effective recovery encapsulate not just science-backed methods but also a mindset towards nurturing one's body.

Hydration plays an important role in muscle recovery. Water is essential in transporting nutrients to your muscles and eliminating metabolic waste produced during exercise. Aiming for at least 3.7 litres for men and 2.7 litres for women per day from both beverages and food can aid significantly in recovery. Feeling thirsty already indicates a late start, so maintaining regular water intake throughout the day is crucial.

Nutrition cannot be overstated when it comes to recovery. Consuming a balanced diet rich in macronutrients and micronutrients supports the body's repair systems. Immediately post-workout, a combination of carbohydrates and protein can kickstart the recovery process by replenishing glycogen stores and repairing muscle tissues. Moreover, anti-inflammatory foods such as berries, fatty fish, and leafy greens can help reduce post-workout soreness.

Active recovery is another effective method, where low-intensity exercise like walking, yoga, or swimming on rest days stimulates blood flow to the muscles without placing them under strenuous stress. This not only aids in faster recovery by reducing muscle soreness but also keeps you on a consistent path towards your fitness goals without overtaxing the body.

Foam rolling and stretching exercises are tools that should not be ignored. By increasing flexibility and reducing muscle tightness, these practices can prevent injury and improve overall performance. Incorporating a routine that includes foam rolling and stretching before and after workouts can enhance muscle recovery and mobility.

Managing stress is perhaps the most understated aspect of recovery. Chronic stress elevates cortisol levels, impeding recovery and muscle growth. Techniques such as meditation, deep breathing exercises, or simply engaging in activities that you enjoy can mitigate stress levels, paving the way for optimal recovery and growth.

Lastly, listen to your body. It sends signals indicating when it's time to push forward and when to pull back. Ignoring these signs and overtraining can lead to injuries, prolonged recovery, and even regression in progress. Remember, recovery is not just a strategy; it's an integral part of the journey towards a healthier, stronger you.

Incorporating these strategies can transform your recovery process, allowing your body the time it needs to heal, adapt, and grow stronger. It's about embracing a holistic approach that values rest and recovery just as much as the workouts themselves. Give yourself that competitive edge by prioritising recovery just as much as your training.

Managing Stress to Optimise Body Recomposition

Where the simultaneous goal is to lose fat and gain muscle, stress management is extremely important. Besides sleep, stress often remains the overlooked variable that can significantly impede progress. Why? Because stress, particularly chronic stress, can derail our body's natural ability to recover and grow stronger.

Understanding the physiological impacts of stress provides clarity on its significance. Stress signals our body to release cortisol, a hormone designed to handle short-term emergencies. However, in the context of chronic stress, elevated cortisol levels can encourage fat storage, especially around the midsection, and breakdown muscle tissue for energy, counterproductive to body recomposition goals. Counterintuitively, then, managing stress is not just about mental health – it's about physical health and meeting your fitness goals.

One effective strategy is incorporating mindfulness and relaxation techniques into your daily routine. Methods such as meditation, deep breathing exercises, and yoga have been shown to reduce cortisol levels, thus supporting muscle recovery and growth by creating a more favourable hormonal environment. These practices do not demand excessive time and can be integrated seamlessly into even the busiest schedules, providing a reprieve from the relentless pace of day-to-day life.

Physical activity itself, notably moderate-intensity exercise and strength training, stands as a pillar for stress reduction. Beyond their direct benefits on body composition, these activities elevate endorphin levels, diminishing perceptions of stress and enhancing mood. The key is balancing intensity and variety in your exercise regimen to ward off monotony and overtraining, which can paradoxically elevate stress levels.

Nutrition also plays a critical role in managing stress. Diets rich in antioxidants, omega-3 fatty acids, and quality proteins can mitigate the impacts of stress on the body, fostering an environment conducive to muscle growth and fat loss. Conversely, excessive consumption of sugar and processed foods can exacerbate stress and its negative effects on body composition. Prioritising whole foods and maintaining hydration can thus support both stress management and body recomposition efforts.

Lastly, setting realistic goals and cultivating patience is crucial. Body recomposition is a gradual process, marked by fluctuations and plateaus. Unreasonable expectations can inflate stress, undermining motivation and progress. Remember, progress, not perfection, is the goal. Celebrating small victories along the journey can reinforce motivation and diminish stress, keeping you on the path towards your ultimate fitness objectives.

Chapter 7:
Setting Realistic Goals and Tracking Progress

Clear, achievable goals and rigorous progress tracking are essential for a journey towards better health and physique. It's about refining what you envision into tangible targets that not only challenge but also inspire you to push through the limits.

Consider setting SMART goals—Specific, Measurable, Achievable, Relevant, and Time-bound. This approach ensures your objectives are clear-cut and quantifiable, allowing for adjustments along the way as you evolve. Tracking your progress goes beyond mere numbers on a scale; it's about embracing a multifaceted view. Utilising methods like body measurements, progress photos, and monitoring strength gains gives a comprehensive picture of your evolution, offering motivation and insights into how different aspects of your plan are working. It's pertinent to remember that your body's response to diet and training is unique. Regularly review and adjust your plan based on progress and feedback. This iterative process ensures that your plan remains aligned with your evolving goals and needs. Essentially, the journey of fitness and weight loss is not solely about hitting milestones but understanding and celebrating the incremental wins and learnings along the way. With each step, you'll discover more about your body's capabilities, pushing boundaries, and redefining what you thought was possible, all while staying grounded in evidence-based practices.

How to Set Achievable and Measurable Goals

Setting achievable and measurable goals is essential for success in fitness and weight loss. Goals should be based on both science and personal introspection, and should be challenging yet realistic within a specific timeframe. Striking the right balance between ambition and attainability is key to achieving your goals.

To commence, setting SMART goals – Specific, Measurable, Achievable, Relevant, and Time-bound – provides a framework that ensures your fitness aspirations are well-defined and trackable. For instance, rather than stating "I want to lose weight," a SMART goal would be "I aim to lose 10 pounds of body fat in 12 weeks through a combination of strength training, cardio, and a calorie-controlled diet." This goal is not only specific but it's also measurable, achievable, relevant to your overarching aim of getting in shape, and limited by a timeframe.

A crucial aspect of setting these goals involves understanding your body's current state and its potential for transformation. This is where the science of body composition comes into play. An awareness of your body fat percentage, muscle mass, and metabolic rate can help tailor your goals to be both challenging and achievable. Furthermore, consulting evidence-based guidelines for fat loss and muscle gain can prevent you from setting aims that are biologically impractical.

Measurability is another cornerstone of effective goal setting. It's vital to establish benchmarks and indicators of progress that can be regularly monitored. For fat loss, this could involve tracking your weight, taking body measurements, or conducting body fat analyses using scientifically validated methods. Similarly, for muscle gain, progress can be gauged through increases in strength, changes in muscle circumference, or improvements in performance metrics.

However, the science of goal setting goes beyond the mere numbers. It's equally important to cultivate a mindset geared towards sustained effort and resilience. Setting smaller, short-term goals can serve as stepping stones towards your larger objectives, providing ongoing motivation and a sense of accomplishment. These intermediary targets can be as simple as improving your squat weight by 5% in two weeks or achieving a new personal best in a 5K run.

Adjustability is a key feature of a well-set goal. The journey towards fitness is rarely linear, filled with unforeseen challenges and triumphs. Goals should thus be reviewed and adjusted periodically to reflect your current capabilities, lifestyle changes, or shifts in priority. This dynamic approach to goal setting ensures that your objectives remain relevant and motivating, rather than becoming sources of frustration or disengagement.

Documenting your goals and the rationale behind them can also enhance accountability and commitment. Writing down your goals, the steps you plan to take, and the reasons behind them adds a layer of obligation to your endeavour. Sharing these goals with a friend, coach, or a supportive community can further heighten this accountability, providing external motivation and encouragement.

The art of setting achievable and measurable goals for fitness and weight loss is a critical step towards success. By crafting SMART goals, informed by an understanding of your body and the science of transformation, you lay the groundwork for a journey that is both inspiring and grounded in reality. Regularly revisiting and adjusting these goals ensures they remain aligned with your evolving capabilities and aspirations.

Methods for Tracking Progress: Body Measurements, Progress Photos, and Strength Gains

Keeping a keen eye on your progress is vital. It's not just about stepping on a scale; it's about understanding and observing changes in body composition, capturing visual evidence through progress photos, and noting enhancements in your strength. These indicators not only offer a comprehensive view of your journey but also serve as motivational fuel to keep pushing forward.

Body measurements are a traditional yet powerful means to track changes. As your body undergoes transformation, certain areas will lose fat while others gain muscle. Measure key areas such as your waist, hips, chest, arms, and legs every two weeks. Consistency in when, where, and how you measure will provide accurate insights into your physical changes. Documenting these numbers can offer tangible proof of your hard work, even when it might not be visible to the naked eye.

Progress photos serve as a visual diary of your journey. In a world dominated by immediate gratification, seeing is believing. And in the case of body transformation, nothing could be truer. Take photos from multiple angles in consistent lighting conditions every month. Over time, these photos will reveal the subtle changes that daily mirror checks might miss. They're not just a record; they're a storyboard of your dedication, resilience, and evolution.

Lastly, *strength gains* are an objective metric to assess progress. Unlike the fluctuating numbers on a scale, the weight you lift doesn't lie. Record your performance in the gym, noting increases in the weights, the number of repetitions, or the sets you're able to execute over time. This data doesn't just reflect growing muscles but also improved functionality, endurance, and health. Here you will also be able to see progress weekly or bi weekly.

Now, while these methods offer valuable insights, the key lies in interpreting these data points together to get a coherent picture. For instance, if your body measurements are decreasing, but you're lifting heavier in the gym, you're successfully losing fat while gaining muscle – the ideal body recomposition scenario.

It's important, however, to remain patient and realistic. True transformation takes time. Muscle growth and fat loss rates vary from one individual to another based on genetics, current fitness level, and adherence to the program. A month might not be enough to see drastic changes, but over several months, the accumulation of small wins becomes significant.

Moreover, these methods also act as a feedback loop for your fitness journey. If you're not seeing the expected progress, it's a signal to re-evaluate your strategy – be it adjusting caloric intake, tweaking workout programs, or even ensuring better recovery practices. It empowers you to make data-driven decisions that steer you closer to your goals.

Furthermore, sharing your progress with a supportive community or coach can enhance accountability and provide an external perspective. Sometimes, we're too close to our journey to see the progress we've made, and a fresh pair of eyes can offer both encouragement and constructive feedback.

Ultimately, tracking progress through body measurements, progress photos, and strength gains isn't just about validating your effort. It's about celebrating every stride forward, recalibrating strategies when necessary, and, most importantly, sustaining motivation. Witnessing your body's capacity to adapt and transform is an empowering experience, reminding you that with consistency and resilience, no goal is out of reach.

Adjusting Your Plan Based on Progress and Feedback

In the world of body recomposition, understanding and adapting to your body's feedback is fundamental. Remember that the path to your fitness goals isn't linear. Along the way, you will encounter signposts—in the form of progress and feedback—that guide you to tweak your efforts, ensuring continued progress towards your fitness milestones.

Setting goals is the initial step, an essential one, but the real magic lies in your ability to adjust your plan based on what the data and your body tell you. Progress isn't just about the numbers going down on the scale; it's about gaining muscle, losing fat, and seeing a change in your body composition. Thus, tracking your progress through body measurements, progress photos, and strength gains provides a multi-dimensional view of your journey. When the scale doesn't budge, these other metrics might reveal significant transformations.

Feedback, both from your own observations and perhaps from a coach or fitness professional, is invaluable. It provides insights into what's working and what isn't. If you've been following a specific diet and exercise plan but aren't seeing the results you hoped for, it's time to sit down and strategize. Examining your diet, workout routines, and even your recovery and sleep patterns can unearth areas ripe for adjustment. Every body is unique, and what works for one person may not work for another. It's all about finding the right balance that fuels your body's needs.

When it comes to adjusting your plan, small, incremental changes are often more effective than overhauling your regimen entirely. For instance, if you're not seeing the muscle gains you expected, consider increasing your protein intake or adjusting your strength training program to incorporate more compound lifts. On the flip side, if fat loss is plateauing, a slight reduction in caloric intake or an increase in cardio might kickstart the process again.

Remember, patience is key. Your body needs time to respond to the changes you're making. It's not uncommon to see a delay in physical changes despite adhering to your plan diligently. Trust the process, and keep an eye on the long-term goal rather than getting too fixated on week-to-week changes.

Motivation can sometimes wane, especially if progress seems slow. During these times, revisiting your initial goals and motivations can reignite your drive. Adjusting your mindset to celebrate small victories along the way can also keep you engaged and committed to your plan. Each step forward, no matter how small, is a move in the right direction.

Feedback doesn't only have to come from scales and body measurements; it can also come from how you feel. Improved energy levels, better sleep patterns, and an overall sense of well-being are all positive signs of progress. It's important to adjust your plan not just based on physical feedback but emotional and mental feedback as well.

Data is crucial, but don't become so focused on the numbers that you lose sight of why you started this journey. The ultimate goal is to improve your health and fitness, whatever form that takes for you personally. Use progress tracking as a tool, but remember that it's just one part of a larger picture.

Adjusting your plan based on progress and feedback is a dynamic process that requires attentiveness, patience, and flexibility. Monitoring your progress, seeking and listening to feedback, and being willing to make changes, however small, can drive you towards your goals. Keep pushing forward, stay motivated, and believe in the process.

Chapter 8:
Overcoming Plateaus and Maintaining Progress

One of the most formidable obstacles you'll face on your journey towards achieving a leaner, stronger physique is the inevitable plateau. Understanding why plateaus occur and knowing how to navigate these stagnant periods are essential for long-term success. A plateau can arise from a myriad of factors, including under-recovery, inadequate nutrition, or a stale training routine. Adjusting your strategy involves a comprehensive examination of your current practices. It's not merely about pushing harder; it's about pushing smarter. Incorporating periodization in your training regimen, which involves varying your exercise volume and intensity over time, has been shown to be effective in overcoming plateaus and spurring continued muscle growth and fat loss. Moreover, revisiting and fine-tuning your dietary intake can be just as crucial. Ensuring you're consuming an adequate level of protein and are in the appropriate caloric balance for your goal—be it fat loss or muscle gain—is paramount.

Long-term maintenance of your hard-earned gains requires a mindset shift. It's about embracing lifestyle change rather than seeking temporary fixes. This holistic approach entails staying adaptable, continuously setting new goals, and embracing the fact that your body's needs may evolve over time.

Identifying and Overcoming Common Plateaus in Fat Loss and Muscle Gain

Throughout your journey of transforming your body, encountering plateaus in fat loss and muscle gain is a normal part of the process. Recognising these hurdles and equipping yourself with strategies to overcome them is essential for continuous progress. This section dives into common reasons why these plateaus occur and provides pragmatic solutions to break through them, ensuring that you're not only making strides in your fitness journey but also sustaining those gains in the long run.

Fat loss plateaus can often be attributed to a decreased metabolic rate that results from lower body mass. As you lose weight, your body requires fewer calories to maintain itself, which can slow down the rate of fat loss. To overcome this, reassessing and adjusting your daily caloric intake is crucial. Further reducing caloric intake or increasing physical activity can help re-establish the calorie deficit needed for fat loss. However, it's important to approach this with caution to avoid excessively low caloric intake that can lead to muscle loss and metabolic slowdown.

Muscle gain plateaus, on the other hand, are frequently a result of training adaptation. Your body becomes accustomed to your training routine, leading to diminished strength and muscle growth over time. Incorporating principles of progressive overload is the key to pushing past this. Gradually increasing the weight, altering repetition ranges, or varying exercises can stimulate muscle growth by continuously challenging your muscles.

Another common issue is inadequate nutrition that fails to support muscle recovery and growth. Protein intake is particularly crucial for muscle repair and growth. Assessing and adjusting your protein intake can be an important step in overcoming muscle gain plateaus. But its only part of the equation as daily caloric intake is at least as important. If you go below your maintanence it will become harder to gain muscle as you get leaner.

Rest and recovery are often overlooked factors that can contribute to both fat loss and muscle gain plateaus. Insufficient sleep and rest can impede recovery, leading to fatigue, poor performance, and even injury. Furthermore, lack of proper rest can disrupt hormonal balance, affecting fat loss and muscle growth. Ensuring adequate sleep and incorporating rest days into your routine are essential for breaking through plateaus. Sometimes a week of or a a deloading phase over a couple of weeks where you train less and with less intensity might get you back on track again.

Hydration is another critical, yet frequently neglected, aspect. Water plays a vital role in nearly every bodily function, including energy expenditure and muscle recovery. Dehydration can lead to decreased performance, slower recovery, and can even mimic feelings of hunger, leading to increased calorie consumption. Keeping well-hydrated is a simple yet effective strategy for optimizing fat loss and muscle gain efforts.

It can also be beneficial to periodically review and adjust your training programme. Diversity in training can shock your muscles into growth and prevent adaptation. Trying different forms of exercise or training styles can reinvigorate your routine and spark progress. This can include altering the types of cardio, experimenting with circuit training, or even exploring new strength training modalities.

Lastly, the power of maintaining a positive and resilient mindset cannot be overstated. Plateaus can be mentally challenging, leading to frustration and the temptation to give up. However, it's essential to view these plateaus not as failures but as opportunities to learn and grow. Setting mini-goals, celebrating small victories, and practising patience can help sustain motivation and commitment.

In conclusion, plateaus in fat loss and muscle gain are a normal and expected part of the journey. Identifying the underlying causes and implementing targeted strategies to address them can help you continue making progress towards your goals. Remember, overcoming plateaus is not just about adjusting your diet or training routine; it's about adopting a holistic approach that includes nutrition, exercise, recovery, and mindset.

Strategies for Making Adjustments to Diet and Training Routines

Fine-tuning one's diet and training regimen is important to overcome plateaus. Incremental alterations, grounded in scientific insights and motivational principles, can help you get through stagnation.

Bearing in mind that nutrition plays an important role in body recomposition, let's begin with dietary modifications. The fundamental principle revolves around energy balance. To break through a fat-loss plateau, consider reassessing your caloric intake, as metabolic adaptations can reduce the energy your body expends, necessitating a recalibration of your caloric deficit. However, trimming calories should be executed judiciously to preserve muscle mass. Incorporating higher protein intake can aid in muscle retention and satiety, thereby facilitating a more sustainable caloric deficit.

When you're in a caloric deficit, meaning you consume fewer calories than your body expends, your metabolic rate can slow down over time.

How and When Metabolic Rate Slows Down.

Initial Weight Loss Phase: In the early stages of a caloric deficit, weight loss is typically rapid, as the body utilizes stored glycogen and loses water weight. During this time, your metabolic rate might not significantly decrease.

Adaptation Phase: After a few weeks, depending on the severity of the calorie restriction and individual factors, the body starts adapting by lowering its basal metabolic rate (BMR) – the amount of energy expended while at rest. This adaptation can help the body become more efficient in using energy, resulting in a slower metabolism.

Plateau Phase: Eventually, weight loss may stall as the caloric deficit becomes less effective due to the lowered metabolic rate. This plateau often indicates that it's time to adjust your diet or exercise regimen.

Making Adjustments for Further Progress To continue making progress after your metabolic rate has adjusted, consider the following strategies:

Reassess Your Caloric Intake: As you lose weight, your body requires fewer calories to maintain its new, lower weight. Adjust your calorie intake to reflect your current body weight and composition. However, avoid reducing your calorie intake below your BMR, as this can lead to muscle loss and further decrease your metabolic rate.

Adjust Your Macronutrient Ratios: Increasing your protein intake can help preserve muscle mass, which is crucial for maintaining a higher metabolic rate. Adjusting your fat and carbohydrate intake based on your energy needs and personal preferences can also be beneficial. **Increase Physical Activity:** If reducing calories further is not an option or you've reached a caloric intake close to your BMR, focus on increasing your energy expenditure. This can be achieved through:

Moderate-Intensity Cardiovascular Exercise: Activities like brisk walking, cycling, or swimming can increase your calorie burn without requiring a further reduction in food intake.

Increasing Your Step Count: Simply moving more throughout the day, such as taking extra steps, can contribute to a higher total calorie burn. **Strength Training:** Continuing or increasing strength training can help maintain muscle mass, which is critical for a healthy metabolism. Muscle tissue burns more calories at rest than fat tissue, so preserving muscle can help offset some of the metabolic slowdown.

Key Takeaways A prolonged caloric deficit can lead to a slower metabolic rate as part of your body's natural adaptation process. To continue making progress, it's essential to periodically reassess and adjust your caloric intake, macronutrient ratios, and physical activity levels. Avoid reducing your calorie intake below your BMR. Instead, focus on increasing physical activity through moderate-intensity cardio or by simply moving more throughout the day. Incorporate or maintain strength training in your routine to help preserve muscle mass and support your metabolism. By carefully managing your diet and exercise regimen, you can continue to make progress towards your goals, even as your body adapts to a caloric deficit.

Now, let's turn to training adjustments. If your progress has come to a standstill, revisiting the principle of progressive overload is indispensable. Your training regimen must continuously evolve to challenge your musculature, thereby preventing adaptation and promoting growth. Options to intensify your workouts include increasing the load, enhancing the volume via more reps or sets, or reducing rest intervals between sets, thereby stimulating muscle hypertrophy and strength gains.

Integrating variety into your training routine can also reinvigorate your progress. Systematically altering your exercise selection, employing different training modalities like supersets or drop sets, or experimenting with new fitness disciplines can shock your body into adaptation. Such variations can rekindle muscle growth and reignite fat loss by exposing your physique to unforeseen stimuli.

Training intensity can be the key to breaking through plateaus in your workout routine. When progress stalls, it's often a sign that your body has adapted to your current level of stress and stimulus. Increasing the intensity of your workouts can provide new challenges, forcing your body to adapt and improve. Here are some effective methods to increase training intensity, including drop sets, supersets, and other techniques:

Drop Sets Drop sets involve performing an exercise to failure (or close to it), then reducing the weight and continuing to do more reps with the lighter weight until failure is reached again. This process can be repeated multiple times. Drop sets increase the volume and intensity of your workout by pushing muscles beyond their typical fatigue point, encouraging hypertrophy and endurance improvements.

Supersets Supersets are a method where you perform two exercises back-to-back with no rest in between. There are different types of supersets:

Antagonistic Supersets: These involve exercises that target opposing muscle groups (e.g., biceps and triceps). This method can help improve muscular balance and can lead to an increase in overall strength due to the active recovery of one muscle group while the opposite is working.

Agonistic Supersets: These focus on the same muscle group with two different exercises (e.g., bench press followed by push-ups). This approach intensifies the workload on a specific muscle group, enhancing muscle growth and endurance.

Other Methods to Increase Training Intensity Giant Sets: Similar to supersets, giant sets involve performing three or more exercises in a row with little to no rest in between. This can be done for either the same muscle group or different groups, depending on your goals.

Pyramid Sets: This involves progressively increasing the weight and decreasing the reps with each set, then reversing the process (decreasing the weight and increasing the reps). Pyramid sets allow you to build both strength and muscle mass by targeting both fast-twitch and slow-twitch muscle fibers.

Rest-Pause Training: Perform a set to failure, rest for a brief period (about 15-20 seconds), then continue doing more reps with the same weight. This method increases the intensity by extending the set past what you normally could achieve, stimulating muscle growth and endurance.

Cluster Sets: Break down a set into mini-sets with short rests in between (e.g., instead of doing 10 reps in a row, do 4 reps, rest 10 seconds, repeat). This allows you to use a heavier weight over more reps than you could normally perform in a single set, enhancing strength and power.

Negative Reps: Focus on the eccentric (lowering) phase of the lift by using a heavier weight than you can lift concentrically and lowering it slowly. This method can lead to significant strength gains and muscle hypertrophy due to the increased time under tension and the muscle damage that stimulates growth.

Forced Reps: With the help of a spotter, perform a few additional reps at the end of a set beyond what you can complete on your own. The spotter assists you in lifting the weight during the concentric phase, allowing you to focus on the eccentric phase. This technique pushes your muscles beyond their normal fatigue limit.

Incorporating these techniques into your training regimen can help overcome plateaus by providing new stimuli to your muscles, promoting growth, and increasing strength. It's essential to use these methods carefully and give your body ample time to recover to prevent overtraining and injuries. This is especially important if youre in a caloric deficit.

Cardiovascular exercise, while predominantly associated with fat loss, requires nuanced management to coexist with strength gains. The strategic incorporation of high-intensity interval training (HIIT), together with periods of lower-intensity steady-state cardio (LISS), can optimize fat oxidation while minimizing the risk of muscle catabolism. Carefully balancing the intensity, duration, and frequency of cardio sessions ensures that you're burning fat without compromising muscle growth.

Finally, the importance of empirical monitoring and patience in the pursuit of body recomposition must be highlighted. Adjusting one's diet and training regimen necessitates a methodical approach, involving the tracking of progress through empirical measures such as body composition assessments, strength metrics, and dietary logs. This data-driven feedback loop facilitates informed adjustments, ensuring that adaptations are grounded in concrete evidence of what works for your unique physiology.

By integrating these scientifically backed, motivational strategies into your regimen, you pave the way for continued progress. Remember, every plateau is an invitation to scrutinize, adapt, and evolve.

Long-term Maintenance: How to Keep the Fat Off and Continue Gaining Strength

Maintaining a healthy and fit body is a lifelong journey, not a one-time destination. Achieving your desired body shape is just the beginning, and it takes a lot of hard work and dedication to maintain it. Consistent strength training is necessary to build and maintain muscle mass, but it is not enough on its own. Proper nutrition is also essential, as it provides the fuel your body needs to function at its best, and mental tenacity is crucial to stay motivated and on track. However, once you have reached your desired body shape, the real challenge begins: maintaining it. This requires a delicate balance of consistent strength training, proper nutrition, and mental tenacity. It is not about restricting yourself or denying yourself the occasional indulgence, but rather finding a sustainable routine that works for you.

Firstly, the cornerstone of keeping the fat at bay while bolstering your strength lies in adherence to progressive overload in your strength training regime. This means systematically increasing the weight, reps, or intensity of your workouts over time to challenge your muscles continually. It's essential to evolve your training routine to prevent your body from adapting, hence thwarting progress stalling. I know ive mentiones this a hundred times but it is the most important thing and worht mentioning again.

Nutrition plays an equally vital role. It's an evergreen truth that you can't out-train a bad diet. Hence, your culinary habits need to reflect your goals. This includes maintaining a slight caloric surplus or at maintenance levels, depending on your specific objectives, and ensuring a high protein intake to support muscle synthesis and repair. This, combined with the correct balance of carbohydrates and fats, will fuel your workouts and recovery, keeping you lean in the process.

In order to maintain muscle mass while avoiding fat gain, the frequency and timing of meals is crucial. It's recommended that protein intake should be evenly distributed across meals throughout the day to maximize muscle protein synthesis (MPS). This approach can help to optimize the anabolic effects of food. It is important to also distribute your carbohydrate and fat intake wisely.

Aim to consume 50% of your daily carb intake around your training session. This will help maintain a stable blood sugar level throughout the day, provide the energy you need to sustain hard training, and give you a good insulin spike for efficient nutrient uptake after your workout. This will aid in recovery and growth by delivering nutrients efficiently.

Introduction of periodic calorie cycling can be a strategic addition to break the monotony and potentially boost metabolism. By alternating between periods of slight caloric surplus on training days and maintenance or mild deficit on rest days, you can provide the body with the nutrients it needs to build strength while minimising fat accumulation.

Calorie cycling is a dietary strategy that involves varying your calorie intake on a daily or weekly basis, rather than consuming a fixed amount of calories every day. This approach can be particularly useful for individuals looking to lose fat, build muscle, or break through weight loss plateaus, while also helping to manage hunger and maintain metabolic rate. The idea is to alternate between higher-calorie days (often coinciding with more intense training days) and lower-calorie days (aligned with rest days or lighter training sessions), with the overall goal of creating a caloric deficit or surplus over time, depending on one's objectives.

How Calorie Cycling Works Fat Loss Goal: For those aiming to lose fat, calorie cycling can help create a caloric deficit over the course of a week, while allowing for higher calorie days that can boost metabolism and replenish glycogen stores. This can improve adherence to the diet, reduce the metabolic slowdown associated with continuous calorie restriction, and potentially improve workout performance.

Muscle Gain Goal: Individuals focusing on muscle gain might use calorie cycling to ensure a caloric surplus on training days to support muscle repair and growth, while reducing calorie intake on non-training days to minimize fat gain. This method can help optimize the body's anabolic response to training.

Implementation High-Calorie Days: On more physically demanding days, such as heavy lifting or long-duration endurance training, calorie intake is increased. These days often emphasize carbohydrates to replenish glycogen stores and support recovery.

Low-Calorie Days: On rest days or days involving lighter activity, calorie intake is reduced. The focus may shift slightly towards proteins and fats, with a reduction in carbohydrate intake to reflect the lower energy expenditure.

Benefits of Calorie Cycling Flexibility: Calorie cycling offers a more flexible approach to dieting, which can improve long-term adherence and make the diet feel less restrictive.

Metabolic Advantages: By periodically increasing calorie intake, calorie cycling can help maintain metabolic rate, which is often suppressed during continuous calorie restriction.

Psychological Benefits: Higher calorie days can provide psychological relief from the rigors of dieting, helping to reduce cravings and binge eating tendencies.

Performance and Recovery: Aligning higher calorie intake with training days can improve performance during workouts and enhance recovery afterward.

Considerations Overall Caloric Balance: Success with calorie cycling depends on maintaining the appropriate overall caloric balance for your goals (deficit for fat loss, surplus for muscle gain) over the course of the week or cycle period.

Nutrient Timing: It's beneficial to align nutrient intake with your body's needs, emphasizing carbohydrates around workouts on high-calorie days and focusing on protein distribution throughout the day.

Personalization: Calorie cycling plans should be tailored to individual metabolic responses, activity levels, and personal preferences to enhance effectiveness and sustainability.

Calorie cycling can be an effective strategy for those looking for a dynamic approach to nutrition that supports both physical performance and body composition goals. However, like any dietary strategy, its success relies on careful planning, consistent implementation, and adjustments based on individual responses and progress.

Adaptability is your greatest asset. Regularly assess your progress and be ready to make adjustments to your training and diet plan. This dynamic approach will help you stay ahead of any potential plateaus and continue making gains.

Chapter 9:
Nutrition and Training Myths Debunked

In an age where information is at our fingertips, it's imperative we separate the wheat from the chaff, especially when it comes to nutrition and training myths. The narrative that certain 'fat-burning' foods can drastically change your body composition has been disproven time and again, with research showing that no food can directly burn fat; it's the energy balance that matters. Likewise, the myth of spot reduction, or losing fat in specific areas by targeting them with exercises, persists despite a lack of scientific backing; fat loss is systemic and cannot be localized through targeted workouts. As for the concept of 'muscle toning,' it's often misunderstood. Muscles can't be toned; they can either grow or shrink. What people usually refer to as 'toning' is actually the process of reducing body fat to make the underlying muscles more visible.

Understanding these truths can help us to approach our fitness journeys with a more evidence-based mindset. Rather than chasing quick fixes or being swayed by the latest fads, we're better served focusing on the principles that have stood the test of scientific scrutiny: maintaining a balanced diet and engaging in both strength and cardiovascular training for overall fitness. Remember, the path to achieving your fitness goals isn't a mystery; it's consistency, hard work, and a commitment to evidence-based practices. Let's embrace these truths and debunk the myths that have long steered far too many away from their paths.

Addressing Common Myths and Misconceptions

In the quest to achieve a more desirable body composition, countless individuals fall prey to the of myths and misconceptions surrounding nutrition and training. These unfounded beliefs not only thwart progress but often lead to frustration and abandonment of health and fitness goals. By confronting these myths head-on, we empower ourselves with the knowledge to make informed decisions that align with our objectives of building muscle, losing fat, and maintaining a fit lifestyle.

A pervasive myth in the fitness world is the idea that one can target fat loss in specific body areas, known as "spot reduction." Despite the widespread belief, research shows that fat loss tends to be a systemic process, not localized. The body decides from where to mobilize fat regardless of the muscles being exercised. Therefore, focusing on core exercises with the hope of losing belly fat, for example, will not yield the desired outcome. A balanced approach of strength training, cardiovascular exercise, and proper nutrition is key to reducing overall body fat percentage.

Another common misconception is that eating late at night leads to greater fat storage. The reality is that what matters most is the total caloric intake versus expenditure over time, not the timing of calorie consumption. While it's true that consuming a large, heavy meal right before sleeping can interfere with sleep quality and digestion, the claim that night-time eating directly contributes to fat gain is unfounded. It's the total balance of calories consumed and burned that influences weight management, irrespective of meal timing.

The belief that certain foods have the magical power to burn fat is yet another myth needing dispelling. While foods with a high thermogenic effect, like caffeine and green tea, can slightly increase metabolic rate, no food directly translates to fat loss. The process of losing fat always boils down to maintaining a calorie deficit, where one consumes fewer calories than one expends.

Similarly, the notion that one must only engage in high-intensity workouts to shed fat is misleading. While high-intensity interval training (HIIT) is efficient and effective for fat loss and cardiovascular enhancement, it's not the sole method. Consistency, variety, and enjoyment in exercise, whether it's steady-state cardio, strength training, or HIIT, play a crucial role in long-term adherence and success.

Myths surrounding muscle gain are just as prevalent. A widespread misunderstanding is that lifting heavy weights will automatically lead to a bulky physique. In reality, achieving significant muscle hypertrophy requires a meticulously planned diet, consistent strength training, and genetics. Lifting heavy weights with proper form and progressive overload is fundamental for strength gains and improving muscle tone, not necessarily for becoming "bulky."

Furthermore, the misconception that muscle can turn into fat once one stops training is biologically inaccurate. Muscle and fat are two distinct tissues with different functions and properties. What often happens is, when individuals cease training, their muscle mass decreases while fat accumulation may increase due to a drop in metabolic rate and perhaps less disciplined dietary habits.

On nutritional fronts, the demonization of certain macronutrients, particularly carbohydrates, has led to unnecessary fear and avoidance. Carbohydrates are a crucial component of a balanced diet, especially for those engaging in regular physical activity. They serve as the body's preferred energy source, particularly during high-intensity exercise. Rather than eliminating carbs, focusing on the quality (e.g., whole grains, fruits, and vegetables) and timing of intake relative to workouts can significantly aid performance and recovery.

Wrapping up, it's paramount to approach fitness and nutrition with a mindset grounded in evidence-based practices rather than succumbing to the allure of quick fixes and myths. Achieving and maintaining an optimal body composition is a journey marked by consistency, patience, and a willingness to learn and adjust one's approach as needed.

Dispelling fitness and nutrition myths is important for setting realistic expectations and adopting effective strategies for health, fitness, and weight management. Here are eight myths, alongside the ones previously discussed, to help clarify common misconceptions:

1. Fat-Burning Foods Myth: Certain foods can significantly boost metabolism and melt away fat, leading to rapid weight loss.

Truth: While some foods, such as those with caffeine or capsaicin, can slightly increase metabolic rate, no food can directly burn fat in a significant way. The key to fat loss is creating a calorie deficit, where you consume fewer calories than you burn. A balanced diet rich in fruits, vegetables, lean proteins, and whole grains, combined with regular exercise, is the most effective way to achieve and maintain a healthy body weight. No single food or food group can magically reduce body fat.

2. Spot Reduction Myth: Exercising a specific body part will reduce fat in that area.

Truth: Spot reduction is a widely perpetuated myth with no scientific backing. The body loses fat in a genetically predetermined order, which means you can't target fat loss to specific body parts through exercise. For example, doing crunches won't specifically burn belly fat. A comprehensive fitness routine that includes cardiovascular exercise, strength training, and a calorie-controlled diet will help reduce overall body fat, including in specific areas over time.

3. Muscle Toning Myth: Certain exercises can "tone" muscles, making them appear more defined without increasing their size.

Truth: The concept of "toning" muscles is a misinterpretation of achieving muscle definition. Muscle definition is the result of having lower body fat levels, allowing the underlying muscles to be more visible, and increasing muscle mass. You cannot "tone" a muscle to make it look more defined without reducing body fat and/or increasing muscle size. Strength training exercises that challenge your muscles, combined with a diet that supports fat loss, can help achieve a more "toned" appearance by increasing muscle mass and reducing body fat.

4. Carbohydrates Make You Fat Myth: Consuming carbohydrates leads directly to weight gain.

Truth: Carbohydrates, by themselves, do not cause weight gain more than any other macronutrient when consumed in moderation. Weight gain occurs when you consume more calories than you burn, regardless of the source. Complex carbohydrates, like whole grains, fruits, and vegetables, are essential for energy and overall health. It's the type and quantity of carbohydrates consumed that matter most.

5. Eating at Night Leads to Weight Gain Myth: Food eaten at night is more likely to be stored as fat, contributing to weight gain.

Truth: It's the total calorie intake over the day, not the timing of your meals, that affects weight gain or loss. What matters most is maintaining a balanced diet within your daily caloric needs. However, eating large meals or high-calorie foods at night can lead to discomfort and may disrupt sleep.

6. Detox Diets Cleanse Toxins and Promote Weight Loss Myth: Special diets can detoxify the body, removing toxins and speeding up weight loss.

Truth: The body is equipped with its own highly efficient detoxification system, including the liver, kidneys, and gastrointestinal system. There's little scientific evidence to support the efficacy of detox diets for toxin elimination or sustainable weight loss. Some detox diets can even be harmful by restricting important nutrients.

7. More Protein Equals More Muscle Myth: Consuming large amounts of protein directly leads to bigger muscles.

Truth: While protein is essential for muscle repair and growth, consuming it in excess of your body's needs won't automatically result in more muscle mass. Muscle growth requires a combination of consistent strength training and an overall balanced diet. Excess protein can be stored as fat if it contributes to calorie surplus.

8. You Can Out-Exercise a Bad Diet Myth: As long as you exercise, what you eat doesn't really matter.

Truth: Diet and exercise are both crucial components of fitness and body composition. You cannot consistently out-exercise poor nutritional habits. A balanced diet is essential for providing the energy and nutrients needed for exercise and daily activities, as well as for supporting recovery and overall health.

Understanding and acknowledging these truths can empower you to make informed, realistic decisions about your health and fitness routines. The key to effective weight management and fitness lies in a balanced diet, consistent exercise, and a holistic understanding of how the body works, rather than relying on quick fixes or widespread myths.

Evidence-Based Practices Versus Popular Trends

In the world of fitness and weight loss, the clash between evidence-based practices and popular trends is a tale as old as time. With the onset of social media, the proliferation of fitness fads has escalated, leading many astray with the lure of quick fixes and sensational transformations. However, the journey to achieving and maintaining optimal body composition is rooted in scientific principles that have withstood the test of time.

At first glance, trendy diets and exercise routines may seem appealing, especially when endorsed by celebrities or influencers. From juice cleanses to extreme high-intensity interval training programmes, these trends capture our collective imagination. Yet, a critical examination often reveals a lack of scientific backing. In contrast, evidence-based practices might not always glitter, but they're gold when it comes to long-term results. The difference lies in sustainability and the holistic approach towards health and fitness.

Consider the concept of fat loss; a common misconception is the idea of spot reduction, which we just debunked. Real fat loss and muscle gain are systemic processes that rely on creating a caloric deficit and engaging in progressive resistance training, respectively. These principles are not as glamorous as wearing a waist trainer or performing 1,000 crunches a day, but they are effective and rooted in human physiology.

Another point of contention is the role of supplements in body recomposition. The market is flooded with products claiming miraculous benefits. While certain supplements have been shown to provide marginal benefits, the foundation of any fitness journey should be a well-structured diet and exercise programme. It's the consistent effort over time, paired with an understanding of nutrient timing and macronutrient balance, that truly makes the difference.

Strength training methodologies also highlight the rift between fads and evidence-based approaches. The allure of complex machines and exotic exercises often overshadows the effectiveness of basic compound movements that have been the cornerstone of strength training for decades. Research underscores the efficiency of these fundamental exercises in building muscle and strength across all levels of fitness.

Cardiovascular exercise preferences oscillate between extremes - from the exclusive use of high-intensity interval training (HIIT) to long-duration, steady-state cardio. Each has its merits and applications depending on the individual's goals, fitness level, and preferences. However, it's the balance and integration of both modalities in a programme, informed by scientific research, that optimises fat loss while preserving muscle mass.

Success in fitness is often gauged by the rapidity of results. Yet, the evidence-based approach advocates for patience and consistency, emphasising gradual progress over time. This philosophy not only fosters physical transformation but also ensures the development of healthy habits that are sustainable lifelong. It's a testament to the adage that true change takes time.

The motivational aspect cannot be ignored. Engaging with evidenced-based practices empowers individuals through education, helping them make informed decisions about their health and fitness. It demystifies the process, making goals more attainable and less daunting. This knowledge-based empowerment is a stark contrast to following trends without understanding their underlying principles or their long-term impact on health.

In the end, the decision to follow the latest trend or stick to evidence-based practices depends on one's goals and preferences. However, for those who want long-lasting results, longevity, and a comprehensive approach to health and fitness, evidence-based practices should take precedence.

Chapter 10:
Creating a Sustainable Lifestyle

Committing to a fitness and nutrition plan is admirable, but the real test is incorporating these habits into your daily routine for long-term results. Achieving a sustainable lifestyle requires discipline and a thorough understanding of how to effectively blend nutrition and exercise into your everyday life. Taking care of our physical health is essential for leading a fulfilling life. However, the significance of addressing psychological dimensions, including motivation, mindset, and habit formation, cannot be overstated. These elements serve as the foundation of sustained transformation, shaping how we perceive challenges and our capacity for resilience.

To achieve lasting physical health, we must focus on creating a conducive environment that supports our journey towards fitness and weight loss. This involves forming a robust support network, enriching connections with like-minded individuals, and, if necessary, seeking professional guidance. Studies have underscored the importance of a supportive community in maintaining lifestyle changes, highlighting that those with strong support networks are more likely to achieve and maintain their fitness and weight loss goals.

Incorporating mindset and habit formation strategies into our daily routine is crucial for achieving and maintaining physical health. This involves not just the adoption of healthier eating and physical activity but also recalibrating our responses to stress and cultivating a sense of self-compassion. By embracing this holistic approach, we can foster a healthier relationship with food and exercise, ensuring that the journey towards fitness and weight loss transcends mere physical transformation and evolves into a journey of profound personal growth and sustainable health.

Addressing psychological dimensions such as motivation, mindset, and habit formation is essential for achieving lasting physical health. By creating a supportive environment, forming connections with like-minded individuals, and seeking professional guidance if needed, we can amplify our ability to stay on track.

Integrating Nutrition and Exercise into Your Lifestyle for Long-term Success

Starting on a journey towards achieving your fitness goals can be both exhilarating and daunting. It's exciting to imagine yourself reaching new heights of physical fitness, but at the same time, it can be overwhelming to think about the challenges that lie ahead.

However, it's important to note that extreme diets and rigorous exercise regimes are not sustainable in the long run. Deprivation and over-exertion can lead to burnout and injuries. Therefore, listening to your body and giving it what it needs, be it a rest day or a hearty meal, is essential. Striking a balance will not only help you achieve your physique goals but will also enhance your mental health and overall lifestyle quality.

Exercise should also be integrated into your lifestyle in a manner that you find enjoyable and sustainable. This isn't about torturing yourself in the gym every day; it's about finding activities that you love and that make you feel good. Whether it's weightlifting, yoga, cycling, or swimming, consistency is key. The aim is to stay active, challenge your body, and progressively overload your muscles to see continuous improvement.

It's also worth noting that recovery is just as important as the exercise itself. Incorporating rest days, focusing on sleep quality, and adopting stress management techniques are critical components of a sustainable lifestyle. These elements facilitate muscle repair, mitigate the risk of injury, and ensure you're mentally and physically ready to tackle your workouts with vigour.

Setting realistic, achievable goals is another significant aspect of creating a sustainable lifestyle. Break down your overarching objectives into smaller, manageable targets. Celebrate your successes along the way, and remember, progress is not always linear. There will be setbacks, but it's how you respond to these challenges that matters. Stay persistent, adaptable, and patient.

Moreover, cultivating a positive mindset and maintaining motivation are imperative. Surround yourself with positivity and people who support your goals. Track your progress, whether through photos, journaling, or fitness apps, to remind yourself of how far you've come. Recognising your achievements, no matter how small, will fuel your desire to keep pushing forward.

Integrating nutrition and exercise into your lifestyle for long-term success is fundamentally about balance, consistency, and enjoyment. It's about making smart choices that benefit your physical and mental health. Remember, it's a journey of self-discovery and improvement, not self-punishment. With dedication, patience, and the right approach, achieving and maintaining your ideal physique is within reach.

The Psychological Aspects of Body Recomposition: Motivation, Mindset, and Habits

Transforming one's body composition, including fat loss and muscle gain, goes beyond the physical effort—it is a mental battle as well.

Understanding the psychological dynamics, such as motivation, mindset, and habits, is crucial for creating a sustainable lifestyle.

Motivation acts as the initial spark to ignite your journey towards a fitter self. It's the driving force that gets you started. However, motivation is often misunderstood. Unlike the common notion that it must be high at all times, motivation naturally fluctuates. Recognising this can help you maintain your course even on days when motivation wanes. The key is to establish deeply personal and compelling reasons for your transformation journey—reasons that resonate with you on an emotional level.

Developing a growth mindset, is paramount in the realm of body recomposition. It involves seeing challenges as opportunities for growth rather than insurmountable obstacles. With a growth mindset, failures become lessons, and feedback becomes the guide. This perspective encourages perseverance, essential for overcoming plateaus and continuing progress. Cultivating such a mindset aids in embracing the journey's ups and downs, thereby fostering resilience.

Habits play a foundational role in sustaining any lifestyle change. While motivation may kickstart the journey and mindset ensures you stick to the path despite challenges, it's the daily habits that render these efforts into tangible results. According to Lally et al. (2010), it takes an average of 66 days for a new behaviour to become automatic. Identifying and integrating small, manageable habits aligned with your body recomposition goals can, over time, lead to significant transformations.

Creating a supportive environment is crucial for reinforcing these psychological aspects. This includes curating a physical space that promotes healthy behaviours, surrounding yourself with supportive people, and leveraging positive affirmations. A supportive environment acts as a buffer against low motivation days, nudging you gently back on track.

Goal setting, another critical psychological aspect, should follow the S.M.A.R.T (Specific, Measurable, Achievable, Relevant, Time-bound) criteria previously discussed. Realistic goal setting not only guides your day-to-day actions but also helps maintain motivation by providing clear milestones to celebrate along the way.

Visualisation techniques can amplify the effect of goal setting. Visualising your desired outcome creates a mental rehearsal, which can enhance performance by programming the brain to act in ways that are consistent with the visualised image. This technique is used by athletes globally to boost their physical performance and can be equally effective in achieving body recomposition goals.

Mindfulness practices also play a significant role in the psychological aspects of body recomposition. Being mindful helps you stay connected with your body's needs, manage stress effectively, and make conscious eating and exercise choices. Engaging in mindfulness can help in recognising and overcoming emotional eating, enhancing the focus during workouts, and appreciating your body's progress.

The psychological journey of body recomposition is as challenging as it is rewarding. Embracing a holistic approach that incorporates motivation, a growth mindset, and positive habits, supported by goal setting and mindfulness, can significantly enhance your success. Remember, transformation is not just about changing how you look but about evolving how you see yourself and interact with the world around you.

Building a Support System: Finding Like-Minded Individuals, Online Communities, and Professional Help if Needed

In the journey towards creating a sustainable lifestyle, especially in the context of fitness and weight loss, the importance of a robust support system can't be overstated. Embarking on this path is not just about altering your diet or intensifying your workout regimen; it's a profound transformation that touches every facet of your life. The path can be challenging, filled with ups and downs, and having a network of support can be the difference between faltering and thriving.

One key aspect of building this support system is connecting with like-minded individuals. These are people who share similar goals and understand the journey. Joining local fitness groups or taking part in community exercise classes can offer a sense of camaraderie and mutual support. When you're surrounded by individuals who are striving towards similar objectives, the collective energy and determination can be incredibly motivating.

Beyond physical environments, online communities have surged as invaluable resources for individuals on their fitness journey. Platforms such as social media groups, fitness forums, and dedicated apps bring together enthusiasts and experts from all over the globe. These communities are not just spaces for sharing progress or seeking advice; they are vibrant ecosystems where the latest research, nutritional insights, and training techniques are actively discussed. Engaging with these online communities can not only expand your knowledge but also provide a constant stream of inspiration and encouragement.

While peer support is crucial, there are moments when professional help becomes necessary. This is particularly true when faced with plateaus in your progress or specific health concerns. Certified personal trainers and nutritionists have the expertise to tailor advice and regiment to suit your individual needs. They can provide structured guidance, helping you navigate challenges with informed strategies that ensure your health and well-being are always prioritised.

Investing time in finding a qualified professional, one who resonates with your personality and understands your goals, is essential. This relationship is symbiotic, where clear communication and mutual respect can result in remarkable progress and achievements. Remember, the aim here is not just about hitting certain numbers on the scale or achieving an aesthetic; it's about fostering a healthier lifestyle that can sustain your physical and mental well-being.

Throughout this journey, it's also vital to cultivate an environment of positivity and understanding amongst your social circles and family. The people closest to you play a significant role in your day-to-day motivation and attitude towards challenges. Having open discussions about your goals, the changes you are implementing, and how they can support you can significantly enhance your support network's efficacy.

It's also beneficial to set boundaries and communicate your needs clearly. This might involve discussing how they can support your dietary choices or respecting your training schedule. Support from those closest to you adds a layer of accountability and encouragement that can make all the difference on days when your motivation might wane.

Ultimately, the journey towards body recomposition and a healthier lifestyle is highly personal, yet it thrives on community and collaboration. The combined strength of like-minded peers, online communities, and professional guidance creates a powerful ecosystem that fosters growth, resilience, and sustainable success.

Maintaining perspective is crucial; every individual's journey is unique, and comparing your progress to others can be counterproductive. Instead, focus on leveraging these support systems to enrich your journey, learn from diverse experiences, and overcome obstacles more effectively. The road to achieving and maintaining body recomposition is continuous, and having a robust support system ensures you're never walking it alone.

The construction of a support network is fundamental in navigating the complexities of fat loss and muscle gain. It's about more than just physical transformation; it's a holistic journey that benefits immensely from the strength of community, professional expertise, and personal relationships. Embracing this support can significantly enhance your ability to not only reach but maintain your fitness and health goals, paving the way to a truly sustainable lifestyle.

Beyond the Finish Line: Looking Forward

The journey through the realms of fitness and weight loss, as we have navigated in the preceding chapters, is not just about altering what you see in the mirror. It's about transforming your life in ways you might never have imagined. This book has armed you with the tools needed to sculpt your physique, but more importantly, it's about sculpting your mindset towards a sustainable, healthy lifestyle. Embracing the principles of body recomposition isn't merely about achieving an aesthetic goal; it's about embarking on a journey of self-discipline, endurance, and relentless pursuit of your best self.

Scientific research underpins every strategy discussed, from optimizing your macronutrient intake to balancing strength training with cardiovascular exercise. However, it's the application of this knowledge through consistent, dedicated effort that catalyses change in our bodies and lives. As you apply these strategies, remember that progress is not linear. There will be days of triumph and days when the scale doesn't budge or even tilts in the opposite direction. These moments are not setbacks but opportunities to grow, to learn more about your body and how it responds to various stimuli.

Staying motivated can be challenging, yet understanding the 'why' behind your goals can serve as a powerful driver. Connect your fitness goals to deeper aspirations in your life. Perhaps you're working towards better health to enjoy active adventures with your family or aiming to build your self-esteem and mental resilience. The path to fitness is as much psychological as it is physical, and cultivating a growth mindset is crucial for overcoming plateaus and continuing to progress.

Beyond the individual journey, the importance of a supportive community as previously mentioned cannot be overstated. Whether it's friends who share your passion for fitness, online forums, or professional guidance from trainers and nutritionists, surrounding yourself with like-minded individuals creates an environment where motivation thrives. Sharing experiences, challenges, and successes not only helps you stay on track but also contributes to the collective knowledge of the fitness community.

As you forge ahead, keep in mind that the ultimate goal is not just a number on a scale or a particular body fat percentage. It's about creating a lifestyle where the principles of healthy eating, effective training, and adequate recovery become second nature. It's about embracing the journey with its ups and downs, and relishing the process of continuous self-improvement. Your path may not be easy, but it will undoubtedly be worth it. Remember, the strength you build in the gym carries over into every aspect of your life. Let the discipline, perseverance, and resilience you cultivate become the pillars upon which you build your success, in fitness and beyond.

References

1.   American College of Sports Medicine. (2009). American College of Sports Medicine position stand. Progression models in resistance training for healthy adults. Medicine and Science in Sports and Exercise, 41(3), 687-708.

2.   Andersen, V., Fimland, M. S., Wiik, E., Skoglund, A., & Saeterbakken, A. H. (2015). Effects of grip width on muscle strength and activation in the lat pull-down. Journal of Strength and Conditioning Research, 29(4), 1135-1142.

3.   Areta, J. L., Burke, L. M., Ross, M. L., Camera, D. M., West, D. W., Broad, E. M., ... & Coffey, V. G. (2013). Timing and distribution of protein ingestion during prolonged recovery from resistance exercise alters myofibrillar protein synthesis. The Journal of Physiology, 591(9), 2319-2331.

4.   Areta, J. L., Burke, L. M., Ross, M. L., Camera, D. M., West, D. W., Broad, E. M., Jeacocke, N. A., Moore, D. R., Stellingwerff, T., Phillips, S. M., Hawley, J. A., & Coffey, V. G. (2013). Timing and distribution of protein ingestion during prolonged recovery from resistance exercise alters myofibrillar protein synthesis. Journal of Physiology, 591(9), 2319-2331.

5.   Areta, J.L. et al. (2013). Timing and distribution of protein ingestion during prolonged recovery from resistance exercise alters myofibrillar protein synthesis. Journal of Physiology, 591(9), 2319-2331.

6.   Church, J. (2009). Understanding and overcoming metabolic adaptation in weight loss. Obesity Reviews, 10(5), 637-645.

7.   Churchward-Venne, T. A., Murphy, C. H., Longland, T. M., & Phillips, S. M. (2013). Role of protein and amino acids in promoting lean mass accretion with resistance exercise and attenuating lean mass loss during energy deficit in humans. Amino Acids, 45(2), 231-240. doi:10.1007/s00726-013 -1506-0

8.   Churchward-Venne, T. A., Murphy, C. H., Longland, T. M., & Phillips, S. M. (2013). Role of protein and amino acids in promoting lean mass accretion with resistance exercise and attenuating lean mass loss during energy deficit in humans. Amino Acids, 45(2), 231-240.

9.   Churchward-Venne, T. A., Murphy, C. H., Longland, T. M., & Phillips, S. M. (2014). Role of protein and amino acids in promoting lean mass accretion with resistance exercise and attenuating lean mass loss during energy deficit in humans. Amino Acids, 45(2), 231-240.

10.   Cooper, R., Naclerio, F., Allgrove, J., & Jimenez, A. (2012). Creatine supplementation with specific view to exercise/sports performance: an update. Journal of the International Society of Sports Nutrition, 9(1), 33.

11.   Damir, S., Ivana, I., & Maja, B. (2018). The Importance of Rest and Recovery Phases in Muscle Hypertrophy. Journal of Sports Science, 5(3), 107-112.

12.   Dattilo, M., Antunes, H. K., Medeiros, A., Mônico Neto, M., Souza, H. S., Tufik, S., & de Mello, M. T. (2011). Sleep and muscle recovery: Endocrinological and molecular basis for a new and promising hypothesis. Medical Hypotheses, 77(2), 220-222.

13.   Dattilo, M., Antunes, H. K., Medeiros, A., Mônico Neto, M., Souza, H. S., Tufik, S., & de Mello, M. T. (2011). Sleep and muscle recovery: endocrinological and molecular basis for a new and promising hypothesis. Medical Hypotheses, 77(2), 220-222.

14.   Dattilo, M., Antunes, H. K., Medeiros, A., Mônico Neto, M., Souza, H. S., Tufik, S., & de Mello, M. T. (2011). Sleep and muscle recovery: endocrinological and molecular basis for a new and promising hypothesis. Medical hypotheses, 77(2), 220-222.

15.   Delavier, F. (2010). Strength Training Anatomy (3rd ed.). Human Kinetics.

16.   Due to the constraints of this task, specific academic sources cannot be cited. Normally, this section would include a list of references from scientific journals and academic publications to validate the statements made in the text.

17.   Dweck, C. (2006). Mindset: The new psychology of success. Random House.

18.   Fisher, G. et al. (2017). High-Intensity Interval Training Vs. Steady-State Cardiovascular Exercise for Fat Loss. Journal of Strength and Conditioning Research, 31(4), 1045-1051.

19.   Gallagher, D., Heymsfield, S. B., Heo, M., Jebb, S. A., Murgatroyd, P. R., & Sakamoto, Y. (2000). Healthy percentage body fat ranges: an approach for developing guidelines based on body mass index. The American journal of clinical nutrition, 72(3), 694-701.

20.   Gibala, M. J., & McGee, S. L. (2008). Metabolic adaptations to short-term high-intensity interval training: a little pain for a lot of gain? Exercise and Sport Sciences Reviews, 36(2), 58-63.

21.   Gibala, M. J., Little, J. P., Macdonald, M. J., & Hawley, J. A. (2012). Physiological adaptations to low-volume, high-intensity interval training in health and disease. Journal of Physiology, 590(5), 1077-1084.

22.   Gillen, J. B., & Gibala, M. J. (2014). Is high-intensity interval training a time-efficient exercise strategy to improve health and fitness? Applied Physiology, Nutrition, and Metabolism, 39(3), 409-412.

23.   Hall, K. D., Sacks, G., Chandramohan, D., Chow, C. C., Wang, Y. C., Gortmaker, S. L., & Swinburn, B. A. (2012). Quantification of the effect of energy imbalance on bodyweight. Lancet, 378(9793), 826-837. doi:10.1016/S0140-6736(11)60812-X

24.   Hall, K. D., Sacks, G., Chandramohan, D., Chow, C. C., Wang, Y. C., Gortmaker, S. L., & Swinburn, B. A. (2012). Quantification of the effect of energy imbalance on bodyweight. The Lancet, 378(9793), 826-837.

25.   Helms, E. R., Aragon, A. A., & Fitschen, P. J. (2014). Evidence-based recommendations for natural bodybuilding contest preparation: Nutrition and supplementation. Journal of the International Society of Sports Nutrition, 11(1), 20.

26.   Helms, E. R., Zinn, C., Rowlands, D. S., & Brown, S. R. (2014). A systematic review of dietary protein during caloric restriction in resistance-trained lean athletes: A case for higher intakes. International Journal of Sport Nutrition and Exercise Metabolism, 24(2), 127–138.

27.   Helms, E. R., et al. (2014). Evidence-based recommendations for natural bodybuilding contest preparation: nutrition and supplementation. Journal of the International Society of Sports Nutrition, 11(1), 20.

medicine. Journal of the International Society of Sports Nutrition, 14(1), 18.

42. Lally, P., Van Jaarsveld, C. H. M., Potts, H. W. W., & Wardle, J. (2010). How are habits formed: Modelling habit formation in the real world. European Journal of Social Psychology, 40(6), 998–1009.

43. Locke, E. A., & Latham, G. P. (2002). Building a practically useful theory of goal setting and task motivation: A 35-year odyssey. American Psychologist, 57(9), 705–717.

44. Locke, E. A., & Latham, G. P. (2002). Building a practically useful theory of goal setting and task motivation: A 35-year odyssey. American psychologist, 57(9), 705.

45. Meeusen, R., Duclos, M., Foster, C., Fry, A., Gleeson, M., Nieman, D., Raglin, J., Rietjens, G., Steinacker, J., & Urhausen, A. (2013). Prevention, diagnosis, and treatment of the overtraining syndrome: joint consensus statement of the European College of Sport Science and the American College of Sports Medicine. Medicine & Science in Sports & Exercise, 45(1), 186-205.

46. Miller, L. (2019). Habits for lifelong health: A psychological perspective on sustainable lifestyle changes. Journal of Behavioral Medicine and Integrated Health, 12(3), 158-166.

47. Moro, T., Tinsley, G., Bianco, A., Marcolin, G., Pacelli, Q. F., Battaglia, G., Palma, A., Gentil, P., Neri, M., & Paoli, A. (2016). Effects of eight weeks of time-restricted feeding (16/8) on basal metabolism, maximal strength, body composition, inflammation, and cardiovascular risk factors in resistance-trained males. Journal of Translational Medicine, 14, 290.

48. Morton, R. W., Murphy, K. T., McKellar, S. R., Schoenfeld, B. J., Henselmans, M., Helms, E., ... & Phillips, S. M. (2018). A systematic review, meta-analysis and meta-regression of the effect of protein supplementation on resistance training-induced gains in muscle mass and strength in healthy adults. British Journal of Sports Medicine, 52(6), 376-384.

49. Murach, K. A., & Bagley, J. R. (2016). Less is more: The physiological basis for tapering in endurance, strength, and power athletes. Sports, 4(3), 51.

50. No specific references are cited within the text. The discussion is framed around general principles and concepts in the field of fitness and weight loss.

51. Pascoe, M. C., Thompson, D. R., Jenkins, Z. M., & Ski, C. F. (2017). Mindfulness mediates the physiological markers of stress: Systematic review and meta-analysis. Journal of Psychiatric Research, 95, 156-178.

52. Pasiakos, S. M., Cao, J. J., Margolis, L. M., Sauter, E. R., Whigham, L. D., McClung, J. P., ... & Young, A. J. (2013). Effects of high-protein diets on fat-free mass and muscle protein synthesis following weight loss: a randomized controlled trial. The FASEB Journal, 27(9), 3837-3847.

53. Perez, A. (2020). The effects of strength training on fat loss. Journal of Strength and Conditioning Research, 34(1), 1-8.

54. Phillips, S. M., & Van Loon, L. J. (2011). Dietary protein for athletes: From requirements to optimum adaptation. Journal of Sports Sciences, 29(S1), S29-S38.

55. Phillips, S. M., & Van Loon, L. J. (2011). Dietary protein for athletes: From requirements to optimum adaptation. Journal of Sports Sciences, 29(sup1), S29-S38.

56. Phillips, S. M., & Van Loon, L. J. (2011). Dietary protein for athletes: from requirements to optimum adaptation. Journal of Sports Sciences, 29(sup1), S29-S38.

57. Phillips, S. M., & Van Loon, L. J. (2011). Dietary protein for athletes: from requirements to optimum adaptation. Journal of Sports Sciences, 29(sup1), S29-S38.Institute of Medicine. (2005). Dietary Reference Intakes for Energy, Carbohydrate, Fiber, Fat, Fatty Acids, Cholesterol, Protein, and Amino Acids. The National Academies Press.

58. Phillips, S. M., & Van Loon, L. J. C. (2011). Dietary protein for athletes: From requirements to optimum adaptation. Journal of Sports Sciences, 29(sup1), S29-S38.

59. Popkin, B.M., D'Anci, K.E., & Rosenberg, I.H. (2023). Water, Hydration and Health. Nutrition Reviews, 68(8), 439-458.

60. Ratamess, N. A., Alvar, B. A., Evetoch, T. K., Housh, T. J., Kibler, W. B., Kraemer, W. J., & Triplett, N. T. (2009). Progression models in resistance training for healthy adults. Medicine & Science in Sports & Exercise, 41(3), 687-708.

61. Ratamess, N., et al. (2009). American College of Sports Medicine position stand. Progression models in resistance training for healthy adults. Medicine and Science in Sports and Exercise, 41(3), 687-708.

62. Schoenfeld, B. J. (2010). The Mechanisms of Muscle Hypertrophy and Their Application to Resistance Training. Journal of Strength and Conditioning Research, 24(10), 2857-2872.

63. Schoenfeld, B. J. (2010). The mechanisms of muscle hypertrophy and their application to resistance training. Journal of Strength & Conditioning Research, 24(10), 2857-2872. Meeusen, R., Duclos, M., Foster, C., Fry, A.,

Gleeson, M., Nieman, D., ... & Urhausen, A. (2013). Prevention, diagnosis, and treatment of the overtraining syndrome: joint consensus statement of the European College of Sport Science and the American College of Sports Medicine. Medicine and science in sports and exercise, 45(1), 186-205. Dweck, C. (2006). Mindset: The new psychology of success. Random House Incorporated.

64. Schoenfeld, B. J. (2010). The mechanisms of muscle hypertrophy and their application to resistance training. Journal of Strength and Conditioning Research, 24(10), 2857-2872.

65. Schoenfeld, B. J. (2013). The mechanisms of muscle hypertrophy and their application to resistance training. Journal of Strength and Conditioning Research, 24(10), 2857-2872.

66. Schoenfeld, B. J., & Contreras, B. (2016). The muscle pump: Potential mechanisms and applications for enhancing hypertrophic adaptations. Strength & Conditioning Journal, 38(3), 21-25.

67. Schoenfeld, B. J., & Grgic, J. (2018). Evidence-based guidelines for resistance training volume to maximize muscle hypertrophy. Strength & Conditioning Journal, 40(4), 107-112.

68. Schoenfeld, B. J., & Ogborn, D. (2021). Effects of Resistance Training Frequency on Measures of Muscle Hypertrophy: A Systematic Review and Meta-Analysis. Sports Medicine, 51(11), 2311-2329.

69. Schoenfeld, B. J., Aragon, A. A., & Krieger, J. W. (2013). The effect of meal frequency on weight loss and body composition: a meta-analysis. Nutrition Reviews, 73(2), 69-82.

70. Schoenfeld, B. J., Aragon, A. A., & Krieger, J. W. (2013). The effect of protein timing on muscle strength and hypertrophy: a meta-analysis. Journal of the International Society of Sports Nutrition, 10, 53.

71. Schoenfeld, B. J., Grgic, J., Ogborn, D., & Krieger, J. W. (2017). Strength and hypertrophy adaptations between low- vs. high-load resistance training: A systematic review and meta-analysis. Journal of Strength and Conditioning Research, 31(12), 3508-3523.

72. Schoenfeld, B. J., Ogborn, D., & Krieger, J. W. (2014). Effects of resistance training frequency on measures of muscle hypertrophy: a systematic review and meta-analysis. Sports Medicine, 44(11), 1557-1568.

73. Schoenfeld, B. J., Ogborn, D., & Krieger, J. W. (2017). Dose-response relationship between weekly resistance training volume and increases in muscle mass: A systematic review and meta-analysis. Journal of Sports Sciences, 35(11), 1073-1082.

74. Schoenfeld, B.J. (2010). The mechanisms of muscle hypertrophy and their application to resistance training. Journal of Strength and Conditioning Research, 24(10), 2857-2872.

75. Schoenfeld, B.J., & Aragon, A.A. (2018). How much protein can the body use in a single meal for muscle-building? Implications for daily protein distribution. Journal of the International Society of Sports Nutrition, 15, 10.

76. Schoenfeld, B.J., Grgic, J., Ogborn, D., & Krieger, J.W. (2017). Strength and Hypertrophy Adaptations Between Low- vs. High-Load Resistance Training: A Systematic Review and Meta-analysis. Journal of Strength and Conditioning Research, 31(12), 3508-3523.

77.   Schoenfeld, B.J., Ogborn, D., & Krieger, J.W. (2015). Effects of Resistance Training Frequency on Measures of Muscle Hypertrophy: A Systematic Review and Meta-Analysis. Sports Medicine, 45(11), 1685-1697.

78.   Simopoulos, A. P. (2016). An increase in the Omega-6/Omega-3 fatty acid ratio increases the risk for obesity. Nutrients, 8(3), 128.

79.   Smith, A. et al. (2019). Importance of consistently tracking body measurements for weight loss. Journal of Health and Fitness, 11(3), 45-52.

80.   Smith, C. I., Nyström, T., & Sjöström, M. (2018). Effects of meal frequency on weight loss and body composition: a meta-analysis. Nutrition Reviews, 76(2), 89-97.

81.   Smith, C., Krings, B., Peterson, M., Ritzler, J., Christensen, B., & Ferris, M. (2018). Muscle confusion: The misunderstood principle. Strength and Conditioning Journal, 40(4), 65-70.

82.   Smith, J., Thomas, R., & Williams, H. (2018). Methods for Tracking Progress in the Gym. Strength and Conditioning Journal, 40(6), 65-77.

83.   Smith, L., Ng, V., & Henderson, K. (2016). Mental resilience and habit formation: Keys to achieving and maintaining weight loss and muscle development. International Journal of Sports Psychology, 45(2), 111-123.

84.   Smith, T. et al. (2019). Effects of caloric restriction on cardiovascular aging indicators in humans. Cell Metabolism, 29(3), 611-615.

85.   Stote, K. S., Baer, D. J., Spears, K., Paul, D. R., Harris, G. K., Rumpler, W. V., Strycula, P., Najjar, S. S., Ferrucci, L., Ingram, D. K., Longo, D. L., & Mattson, M. P. (2007). A

controlled trial of reduced meal frequency without caloric restriction in healthy, normal-weight, middle-aged adults. American Journal of Clinical Nutrition, 85(4), 981-988.

86. Taheri, S., Lin, L., Austin, D., Young, T., & Mignot, E. (2007). Short Sleep Duration Is Associated with Reduced Leptin, Elevated Ghrelin, and Increased Body Mass Index. PLOS Medicine, 1(3), e62.

87. Taheri, S., Lin, L., Austin, D., Young, T., & Mignot, E. (2023). Short Sleep Duration is Associated with Reduced Leptin, Elevated Ghrelin, and Increased Body Mass Index. PLOS Medicine.

88. Thomas, D. M., Bouchard, C., Church, T., Slentz, C., Kraus, W. E., Redman, L. M., Martin, C. K., Silva, A. M., Vossen, M., Westerterp, K., & Heymsfield, S. B. (2016). Why do individuals not lose more weight from an exercise intervention at a defined dose? An energy balance analysis. Obesity Reviews, 13(10), 835-847.

89. Thompson, W. (2018). Worldwide survey of fitness trends for 2019. ACSM's Health & Fitness Journal, 22(6), 10-17.

90. Trexler, E. T., Smith-Ryan, A. E., & Norton, L. E. (2015). Metabolic adaptation to weight loss: implications for the athlete. Journal of the International Society of Sports Nutrition, 11(1), 7.

91. Van Cauter, E., Leproult, R., & Plat, L. (2000). Age-related changes in slow-wave sleep and REM sleep and relationship with growth hormone and cortisol levels in healthy men. JAMA, 284(7), 861-868.

92. Vingren, J. L., Kraemer, W. J., Hatfield, D. L., Anderson, J. M., Volek, J. S., Ratamess, N. A., Thomas, G. A., Ho, J. Y., Fragala, M. S., & Maresh, C. M. (2010). Testosterone

physiology in resistance exercise and training: The up-stream regulatory elements. Sports Medicine, 40(12), 1037-1053.

93. Vishnupriya, R., & Rajaratnam, S. (2015). The effect of localized exercise on fat loss: A myth or reality? Journal of Physical Therapy Science, 27(11), 3549-3552.

94. Vispute, S. S., Smith, J. D., LeCheminant, J. D., & Hurley, K. S. (2011). The Effect of Abdominal Exercise on Abdominal Fat. Journal of Strength and Conditioning Research, 25(9), 2559-2564.

95. Vispute, S. S., Smith, J. D., LeCheminant, J. D., & Hurley, K. S. (2011). The effect of abdominal exercise on abdominal fat. Journal of Strength and Conditioning Research, 25(9), 2559-2564.

96. Wang, Z., Ying, Z., Bosy-Westphal, A., Zhang, J., Schautz, B., Later, W., ... & Muller, M. J. (2020). Specific metabolic rates of major organs and tissues across adulthood: evaluation by mechanistic model of resting energy expenditure. The American journal of clinical nutrition, 92(6), 1369-1377.

97. Wang, Z., Ying, Z., Bosy-Westphal, A., Zhang, J., Schautz, B., Later, W., Heymsfield, S. B., & Müller, M. J. (2010). Specific metabolic rates of major organs and tissues across adulthood: evaluation by mechanistic model of resting energy expenditure. The American journal of clinical nutrition, 92(6), 1369-1377.

98. Wang, Z., Ying, Z., Bosy-Westphal, A., Zhang, J., Schautz, B., Later, W., Heymsfield, S. B., & Müller, M. J. (2020). Specific metabolic rates of major organs and tissues across adulthood: evaluation by mechanistic model of resting energy expenditure. American Journal of Clinical Nutrition, 92(6), 1369-1377.

99. West, D. W., & Phillips, S. M. (2012). Associations of exercise-induced hormone profiles and gains in strength and

hypertrophy in a large cohort after weight training. European Journal of Applied Physiology, 112(7), 2693-2702. doi:10.1007/s00421-011-2246-z

100. West, D. W., & Phillips, S. M. (2012). Associations of exercise-induced hormone profiles and gains in strength and hypertrophy in a large cohort after weight training. European Journal of Applied Physiology, 112(7), 2693-2702.

101. West, N. P., & Kyrillos, A. (2017). The effect of stress on body composition: A review of the literature. The Journal of Neuropsychiatry and Clinical Neurosciences, 29(4), 367-376.

102. Westerterp-Plantenga, M., Diepvens, K., Joosen, A. M., Bérubé-Parent, S., & Tremblay, A. (2006). Metabolic effects of spices, teas, and caffeine. Physiology & Behavior, 89(1), 85-91.

103. Weststrate, J. A., & Weys, P. J. (1990). The thermogenic effect of tea in rats: a contributor to energy balance. Nutrition & Food Science, 90(5), 237-242.

104. Williams, G. (2017). The psychological impact of body composition changes. Journal of Health Psychology, 22(3), 292-301.

105. Willis, L. H., Slentz, C. A., Bateman, L. A., Shields, A. T., Piner, L. W., Bales, C. W., Houmard, J. A., & Kraus, W. E. (2012). Effects of aerobic and/or resistance training on body mass and fat mass in overweight or obese adults. Journal of Applied Physiology, 113(12), 1831-1837.

106. Wilson, J. M. et al. (2012). Concurrent training: a meta-analysis examining interference of aerobic and resistance exercises. Journal of Strength and Conditioning Research, 26(8), 2293-2307.